"This is a must read for those suffering from chronic illness or caring for someone with health problems. Jeffrey Boyd draws on his years of professional and personal experiences to write this brilliantly clear and easy to read book on how to be truly well even in the midst of sickness and trial. It is packed full of practical insights that will lift your spirit, bring you closer to God, and may even contribute to your healing."

Harold G. Koenig, M.D., codirector, Center for Spirituality, Theology, and Health, Duke University Medical Center

"The most comprehensive and understandable treatise on chronic illness that I have had the pleasure to review. It deals in a very practical way with questions I hear in my office every day. I plan to use this book for my patients. It should be part of the training for all who work with those with a chronic disease, from physicians to social workers. If you or a loved one has a diagnosis of an incurable disease, this book can be immensely helpful and can save you a great deal of time and work in determining the best course of action."

David Podell, M.D., Ph.D., Yale Medical School

"A richly textured portrait of how people live with disease. It is immensely moving. In describing his own odyssey as a caregiver, Boyd displays rare candor and eloquence. This book is about resilience in the face of adversity, a theme that is central to the Bible. It is filled with practical advice. It is well-organized, and written in language that is easy to understand. Boyd's endorsement of optimism is in the best medical tradition, and simultaneously arises from the Bible."

Harold Ellens, Ph.D., author, *God's Grace and Human Health*

"In this remarkable book, Dr. Boyd distills the latest research concerning the increasing amount of chronic illness into easy-to-understand language. Dr. Boyd is a gifted researcher in the field of chronic disease epidemiology. His works have been at the forefront. This book is a labor of love, compassionately written by a caregiver whose wife died of a multitude of chronic diseases. *Being Sick Well* is a wonderful book, gritty, honest, intimate, uplifting and deeply moving."

Darrel Regier, M.D., M.P.H., formerly at the National Institutes of Health

"Guaranteed to make you proud to be simply human! Jeffrey Boyd has interviewed 'experts'—people who live joyfully despite chronic disease—and he shares their stories with compassion, clarity, and humor. With his training as physician and clergyman he provides practical wisdom for living, with a Christian perspective."

Auguste Fortin, M.D., Yale Medical School

"If Martin Luther is right in saying, 'In the teeth of death we live,' Jeffrey Boyd shows how those teeth marks can become healing stripes and our maker's marks."

Leonard Sweet, Ph.D., author,
SoulTsunami, *SoulSalsa*, and *FaithQuakes*

"I suffer from several chronic illnesses. Jeff Boyd has totally changed my life. Here we have a truly remarkable book. Essential reading for all who have a chronic disease. Dr. Boyd's sense of compassion shines through on every page as he illuminates emotional territory with lightning clarity, encourages us not only to heal our wounds, but to use our gifts. *Being Sick Well* is an emotionally intelligent guide to good health and well-being."

Susanna Knoble, Sebring, Florida

BEING
SICK
WELL

Joyful Living Despite Chronic Illness

JEFFREY H. BOYD, M.D., M.P.H.

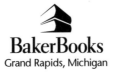

BakerBooks

Grand Rapids, Michigan

Published by Baker Books
a division of Baker Publishing Group
P.O. Box 6287, Grand Rapids, MI 49516-6287

Printed in the United States of America

Library of Congress Cataloging-in-Publication Data
Boyd, Jeffrey H.
    Being sick well : joyful living despite chronic illness / Jeffrey H. Boyd.
        p.   cm.
    Includes bibliographical references.
    ISBN 0-8010-1268-6 (pbk.)
    1. Chronically ill—Religious life. 2. Chronic diseases—Religious aspects—Christianity. I. Title.
    BV4910.B69 2005
    248.8′61—dc22   2004027397

CONTENTS

ILLUSTRATIONS

Figures

Tables

INTRODUCTION

The Trend and How to Cope

My wife, Pat, had two heart attacks and two strokes. She had diabetes, her kidneys failed, and she went on dialysis. She had bypass surgery on her legs, but eventually both were amputated above the knees. Over several decades she went blind and her hands became numb. At age fifty she died.

What kept Pat upbeat despite all this? Three things. First, she was a devoted mother. She was willing to go through anything, provided that our daughter, Felicity, was okay. Second, Pat and I became increasingly spiritual. Medical research shows that spirituality is a powerful resource for dealing with stress. We were devoted servants of Jesus Christ. We prayed often for healing, but God's answer was, "Not yet!" Third, Pat's medical disasters were not her main experience in life. The diseases were often quiet and well behaved. There were long periods of normal life. Even when Pat was on peritoneal dialysis, it became part of the ordinary routine. Life itself was delicious. It was sometimes possible to deny the danger, ignore the illnesses, and simply enjoy the blessings that God sent us in such abundance.[1]

I cannot say that Pat and I were always successful in dealing with her illness. In the end I was humbled, feeling I had not been as good a caregiver as I should have been.

There is an epidemic of chronic illness today. Catherine Hoffman found that 90 million Americans had a chronic illness in 1987.[2] By 1998 that number grew to 120 million, according to Gerard Anderson's research team at Johns Hopkins.[3] At least 45 percent of all Americans have a chronic condition, accounting for 78 percent of the health-care budget.[4] These numbers are increasing. By 2030 the number of Americans with a chronic disease will be 171 million.[5] These are huge numbers. This is the largest epidemic that has ever swept our civilization, bigger than the epidemic of heart disease, cancer, AIDS, and Alzheimer's disease combined, because it encompasses and includes those other epidemics. This epidemic has swept the globe. Every technologically advanced society has the same escalating problem that causes skyrocketing medical costs.

I set about to learn how people had successfully endured the affliction of chronic illness. I asked doctors, nurses, clergy, and other friends to refer to me the name of anyone they knew who had lived with a dreadful illness for a prolonged period of time yet remained upbeat. Then I interviewed those people, learning how they managed to live with a positive attitude. This book contains the wisdom distilled from those interviews. Twice as many women as men were referred to me. I interviewed Protestants, Catholics, Jews, Muslims, Buddhists, Hindus, agnostics, atheists, and those with nonspecific spirituality. They had a range of chronic illnesses or were caring for someone with a chronic illness and came from a wide geographic distribution, from Maine to California to Florida. While many were disabled by their illnesses, others worked full time as a housewife, banker, barber, teacher, software engineer, doctor, chiropractor, lawyer, or minister.

Here is what I found from these interviews: A woman whose child is born with multiple defects is overwhelmed with sorrow. Then her family and friends gather around her, and she feels so supported that the birth defects are seen as a blessing in disguise. Someone with severe lupus and brain tumors uses humor to mock the diseases, allowing her co-workers to laugh with delight, thus preserving dignity and nobility in the face of suffering. Someone with terrible arthritis puts a brown paper bag in the middle of the dining room table at a party. She says that anyone who even mentions her pain that night must put five dollars in the bag. The party is a success because no one discusses her illness. Many people feel closer to God as they endure unavoidable suffering, and that relationship sustains them. These are some of the ways that people live well despite being sick.

Like the Centers for Disease Control (CDC), I define chronic conditions as those that "are prolonged, do not resolve spontaneously, and are rarely cured completely."[6] Many readers misunderstand and think that chronic conditions are devastating illnesses. Doctors and laypeople have different definitions of the term "chronic illness." While devastating illnesses are part of what this book is about, the word *chronic* means "long term." High blood pressure is the most common chronic condition.

This book has two core themes: One theme is that there is an increasing epidemic of chronic illness. Another theme is that some people have lived joyfully despite their chronic illness, and we can learn by listening to them. Like C. S. Lewis, I define *joy* as "moments when you were too happy to speak."[7]

I do not mean to say that joy is always within the reach of sick people. Job in the Bible finds no joy until God rescues him from his skin disease and other catastrophes and restores Job's fortunes. Some people who suffer on this earth will find happiness only in heaven, after they die. Nevertheless, it can be encouraging to read about the minority of sick people who manage, against all odds, to remain happy during this imperfect earthly life.

Although there has been an epidemic of chronic diseases over recent decades, there is not necessarily a progressive increase in the amount of human suffering. Why? Because the diseases are sometimes less devastating than they used to be. We are learning to diagnose them earlier and manage them better.[8] Among the elderly in the United States, there is a decrease in the level of disability.[9] This is not true for younger age groups,[10] but it is true for the elderly.[11] People age sixty-five and older are less disabled today by the same diseases than their grandparents would have been if they had been afflicted with those diseases fifty years earlier. Kenneth Manton was the first to note this decline in the rate of disability among people sixty-five and older.[12]

We learn more from stories of success than from stories of defeat. This is a book about success and how to achieve it. I think it is valid to present in these pages a triumphant minority of sick people who find a way to remain upbeat even during this earthly pilgrimage. This is a book about resilience, courage, spiritual virtues, and the abundance of blessings that healthy people often take for granted.

My goal has been to write a book that sick people will find helpful. My experience is that these stories of successful living provide ideas and motivation for those who feel defeated. The stories inspire them to think of new ways to accept the unacceptable and live with incurable illness. Like the phoenix rising out of the ashes, this book abounds with paradoxes.

In my twenty-five years as a physician, I have spoken with thousands of people who adapted to their chronic diseases, sometimes well, sometimes poorly. Usually people find a way to cope with sickness, not because they want to but because, if it is neither curable nor lethal, what other choice do they have?

Dr. Dennis Dobkin, a cardiologist I know, says, "I always wonder how I would do with a devastating illness. Would I be one of the ones who were crushed, or would I be one of the few who kept my head above water? I fear I would not be able to do it! It is incredible what some people live with, either their own illness or something wrong with their child. Some parents take care of a sick child for fifty years! As a doctor you meet some awesome people, real heroes."

This book will not focus only on sick people. We will focus also on unpaid caregivers, like the parents that Dr. Dobkin mentions. The problems of caregivers are different from those of sick people. It is important that we keep them in mind also. Chapter 8 will especially address caregivers whom I interviewed.

My own chronic illness has been major depression. I inherited it from my father, who had it worse than I. My tendency toward gloom and pessimism has waxed and waned since early childhood. It is insidious. Without realizing it, I drift into the assumption that people are hostile and life is grueling. My tendency toward negativity is the opposite of what is taught in the Bible, which is a book that encourages optimism, because, after all, God triumphs in the end.

I have had a lot of therapy and antidepressant medicines over the years. But the medicine that has helped my disease the most is what I experienced in writing this book. I learned from my teachers—the people I interviewed—how to live a healthier life. Currently I am off all medicines and am exercising every day. I have consciously broadened my commitment to the people who are in my life: my wife, Maureen, and my children, the members of my church, my widowed mother, and my friends. By studying the book that the Lord has assigned me to write, I have learned how to live a happier life. This book is my version of Complementary and Alternative Medicine (CAM), and it's proven to be better than Prozac.

Life sometimes feels like a jumbled chaos. Each person makes meaning of it in a different way. Amidst all the ambiguity and confusion of a long-term disease, some people feel defeated, while others rise to the challenge and lead triumphant lives. Increasingly I think that it is realistic to celebrate life regardless of our circumstances.

Theme One: Being Sick Well

When I talked with people who had a chronic illness but remained upbeat, I discovered that they had developed methods to help them get through each day. I have distilled these methods into twenty strategies, which will be illustrated with case histories throughout the book. Here is a glimpse of what the people I interviewed taught me.

1. Cultivate Your Social Network

People are happier when they have family and friends supporting them than when they feel isolated. In chapter 1 you will meet Sue Sowle, whose son Zachary was born with many birth defects. At first, she was devastated. Now that Zach is five years old, she recalls that her family has supported her.

2. Keep Your Priorities Straight

Parents are sometimes willing to endure any suffering, provided their kids are okay. When you are losing 90 percent of everything because of an illness, it is important to sort out your priorities concerning what 10 percent is worth fighting to preserve. For many people, children or God emerge as the highest priorities. One such person is Suzanne Luchs, whom you will meet in chapter 1. She lives with pain from fibromyalgia, migraines, and endometriosis. She once had a migraine headache that lasted continuously for one year. But she feels that God blessed her because her children (Nora and Jia) are more important than her illnesses.

3. Don't Dwell on Your Illness

People who spend all their time thinking and talking about their sickness tend to feel miserable. It is important to remain engaged with life and keep your illness from eclipsing the many blessings that you still have. Often the best plan is not to talk about it at all, as you will learn from Mary (chapter 1), who chooses to avoid conversation about her arthritis pain.

4. Adopt a Positive Attitude

You can make a conscious decision to take a positive rather than negative approach to life. In chapter 2 you will read about quadriplegics in wheelchairs who play a game called Quad Rugby with exuberance and laughter.

5. Avoid Disaster

Sick people fear three things above all else: (1) impoverishing their families, (2) losing their independence, and (3) becoming a burden to others.[13] Life is better for those who are able to avoid these three disasters. Sharon, in chapter 2, suffers from an unusual case of polio. She fought hard for and won her independence from her parents.

6. Use Humor

Bette Furn (in chapter 3) uses humor to stay in touch with her friends via email while she endures four years of breast cancer treatment. Some sick people and their caregivers ridicule the illness or the callous indifference of healthy neighbors or managed care companies. The humor I've found among sick people is difficult to reproduce. It is often a dark humor, sarcasm, irony, almost a gallows humor. Outsiders sometimes think these remarks are "sick," not funny. Here is an example: Peter Swet, a *People* magazine writer, had a devastating stroke as a young man, leaving him disabled. He wrote a book, *Cracking Up*, about his experiences in a rehabilitation hospital. Normally you would not find it funny to say, *"Nice day for a brain hemorrhage,"* which is the subtitle of his book. But if you read Swet's book, you would find that comment hilarious. My point is that you have to be an insider to appreciate the humor of sick people. Outsiders don't get it. The comment, "Nice day for a brain hemorrhage," captures how vulnerable we are. We may think we live in a secure world when, *wham*, the next minute we are stricken. Often the humor of sick people and their caregivers expresses this meaning: If healthy people had to live with what we live with, they wouldn't believe it. They would say, "This is so grotesque that it can't be happening!"

7. Take One Day at a Time

With illness comes uncertainty about the future. In chapter 3 you will meet Deborah Chase, who has had many heart attacks and strokes. She never knows whether she will be dead or in the intensive care unit tomorrow. Yet she remains cheerful. How? She doesn't think about tomorrow but lives in the present moment. As Jesus says, "Do not worry about tomorrow, for tomorrow will worry about itself. Each day has enough trouble of its own" (Matt. 6:34).

8. Exercise as Much as You Can

Exercise is a cornerstone of health and protection against illness. Walking even prevents Alzheimer's disease.[14] Not only does exercise help prevent the onset of a disease, it slows the progression of disease and promotes a feeling of well-being. My friend Gordon Lewis, a seventy-six-year-old theologian from Denver Seminary, has chronic lung disease. He finds he is able to breathe better and take less medicine when he works out in a gym two times a week. My ninety-year-old mother goes to aerobics two times a week. This practice gives her energy and decreases her aches and pains, though she has had two knee replacements for osteoarthritis. Her neighbor, Mayo Okada, swims every day at age 101. Exercise will be discussed in chapter 4.

9. Use Spiritual Coping

There is an advantage to having a disease! That may sound bizarre, but paradoxically it is true. When an illness whittles you down so you become less self-sufficient, you are less able to rely on your own abilities and more likely to turn to spiritual resources for help. You put fewer eggs in the visible basket of this life and more eggs in an invisible spiritual basket. Though she was blind, Fanny Crosby lived triumphantly and wrote nine thousand hymns in praise of God. In chapter 5 I will demonstrate that the term *spiritual coping* has a wide range of meanings within the religious pluralism of the United States. You will read the case histories of Donna Joblonicky, who has a nonspecific spirituality; Morris Days, who is a Muslim; Jim Koshu, a Buddhist; and Walter Unger, a Christian. All of them use spiritual coping to deal with devastating illnesses. In that chapter, I will introduce some of the medical research that shows spiritual coping helps sick people live well.

10. Say the Jesus Prayer

In chapter 6 I discuss spiritual techniques that come out of the Christian tradition. There is a stress management technique that has been taught in the Eastern Orthodox Church for fifteen hundred years but today every stress management expert I know ignores it. The Jesus Prayer, also known as the Prayer of the Heart, consists of repeatedly saying, "Lord Jesus Christ, have mercy on me!" Even Catholics and Protestants today use this prayer to deal with medical suffering. Compared with relaxation techniques so widely taught in the United States today, this prayer orients us to look for salvation from Jesus, rather than seeking to find it inside ourselves. Tom Powers Jr., better known as "Dooley," in chapter 6, finds in the Jesus Prayer a way to contend with pain, anxiety, and frustration. For years he has endured cancer, as well as heart and bowel disease.

11. Go to Church

Medical research indicates that you live a healthier life if you go to church or a place of worship. Thirty research studies have found that people who attend church, synagogue, mosque, or temple live longer and have more friends (on average) than those who don't.[15] When the tornado of sickness strikes, you are better off if you have a community of people with similar values to support you. An aging couple that moves across the country to live close to their children can usually find a nearby place of worship with a familiar service. If they get sick, their roots in that place of worship can sustain them better than if they had no church, temple, or mosque. In chapter 6 you will read about Charlene Slaver, who has adapted to life with traumatic brain injury and memory deficits. Church plays a crucial role in her ability to cope with these disabilities.

12. Change the World

My brother-in-law, Chris Goffredo, lived with his parents in Stoughton, Massachusetts, when toxic waste seeped through the ground water and contaminated the air in their house with trichloroethane and vinyl chloride. These chemicals got into Chris's bedroom, as in the movie *A Civil Action* with John Travolta. They were absorbed into his body, damaging his immune system so that he became allergic to wheat, gluten, and corn. They also caused a mysterious chronic illness consisting of an array of problems: elevated liver function tests, fragile bones that break, diffuse joint pain, nebulous chest pains, and intermittent collapse of his right leg.

The company that had dumped the chemicals bought the Goffredo house (which was then condemned) and paid money to Chris and his parents for damages. But Chris was left with his mysterious and unnamed chronic disease. As a result of his experience, Chris became an environmental crusader. Working with others, he formed the Stoughton Citizens' Association, which got a grant from the State of Massachusetts. They hired an engineering firm to make surprise inspections of potential polluters and to increase public awareness of the dangers of toxic waste dumped in the environment. They discovered that the town water supply was at risk because chemicals in the ground were inching closer to the reservoir.

When Chris speaks in public, his personal history makes him a compelling advocate for protecting the environment. Becoming a catalyst for change has helped Chris psychologically. For more than a year he was on crutches or in a wheelchair because of broken feet. When his own symptoms persist and he is threatened with the hopeless feeling that nothing will ever change for him, he is comforted by knowing that things will change for other people. In the future, companies won't be able to get away with dumping toxic chemicals, because of the work of the Stoughton Citizens' Association. Strategy 12, Change the World, means letting your chronic illness become your motivation to make a difference. In chapter 6 you will read about Arlene Pond, who uses her disability as a platform for spreading the gospel.

13. Take Charge

Someone must serve as team leader when dealing with the complexities of healthcare. Generally you will get better medical attention if you are the team leader, rather than being passive and hoping that your doctor will take the lead. Walt Larimore uses an analogy of a coach and quarterback on a football team. You can rely on your physician to be your healthcare coach, but you cannot expect the doctor to also be the quarterback. "You need to become your own healthcare quarterback," Larimore writes. "The best teams—the ones that win the most—have great quarterbacks working with great coaches. In your 'health game,' you need to learn how to call the plays."[16] In chapter 7 you will meet Eileen Clarke, who serves as healthcare coach for her two daughters (Kayla and Kelsey) with type I diabetes. At the girls' school, Eileen encourages the teachers and school nurse to treat her daughters as normal kids who just happen to test their blood sugar. She is so skilled at her role that the diabetes becomes a nonissue.

14. Take the Medicine as Prescribed

Richard Geiger knows a lot about how his mind works, because of his Buddhist training in meditation. He finds that his mind works better, that he is happier, when he takes the antidepressant medicine that is prescribed. You will read about him in chapter 7. This is important because research indicates that less than half the pills prescribed by physicians are actually swallowed by patients, which leads to an unnecessary risk of disease flare-up. Among people with high blood pressure, those who take their medicine and avoid having a heart attack or stroke will, of course, be happier. People with a seizure disorder are happier if they have no seizures, because they remember to take the antiseizure medicines. This principle holds for many diseases. People who take the prescribed medicine and are hospitalized three times a decade are happier than those who forget to take the pills and are hospitalized twelve times a decade. This is a strategy that can modify the course of the illness, taming the beast and making it less beastly.

15. Expect a Cure

Many diseases for which there is no treatment today will be curable tomorrow. Remaining optimistic about finding a cure is one way to improve your attitude. Raising money to support research is also uplifting. In chapter 7 you will read about the optimism of my barber, Placido Mastroianni, who expects doctors someday to cure him of the vascular problems that today are incurable. Placido has had a stroke, coronary artery disease, an obstruction to the blood supply of his intestines, and prostate cancer, yet he is exuberant! That's why I have kept returning as his customer over the last thirty years.

16. Keep Busy

There is a natural tendency when you get sick to retreat into your room, close the door, and stay in bed. This is called the "sick role." Such a retreat from life works well when you have a short-term illness but backfires when you have a chronic disease. You can't let life pass you by! You've got to get moving again! Erik Weihenmayer was plunged into darkness at age thirteen by a rare disease called retinoschisis. At age thirty-two he became the first blind person to climb Mount Everest. In chapter 7 I will tell you about Jim Lubin and Brooke Ellison, who live rich lives despite being quadriplegic. In each case the largest muscle the person can control is his or her tongue. All muscles below the neck are paralyzed. Though Jim and Brooke are dependent on respirators to breathe for them, they are actively engaged in life.

17. Take Pride in Your Work as a Caregiver

When medical professionals speak of caregivers, we usually mean those who are paid, like visiting nurses or home health aides. This is a self-centered, narcissistic, and distorted viewpoint for health professionals to have, because the majority of those who care for patients with chronic diseases are unpaid family and friends. There are ten million people in the United States who spend at least twenty-four hours a week taking care of a sick person without pay.[17] Actually the unpaid caregivers are the most important members of the treatment team, but physicians often ignore them. What gives caregivers the strength to keep carrying the heavy burden? One answer is for caregivers to take pride in doing a difficult job well. Beth Brown (chapter 8) says, "I know what God is calling me to do, and I am doing it." Beth leads a quiet life at home, taking care of her husband, Don, who had a stroke years ago. Both Beth and Don were college professors before living the cloistered life that has been forced on them.

18. Enjoy the Blessings

Charlene Stephens (chapter 8) gives another strategy for living with chronic illness. Her daughter, Carla, has brain damage from uncontrolled seizures. For the past sixteen years Charlene has rarely left Carla's side. Carla has no language, is not toilet trained, and is confined to a wheelchair. Although this isn't the life Charlene had imagined for herself, nevertheless, when she learned to live within the constraints of reality, she found life was full of blessings. Charlene and her husband, Bill, have developed a cottage industry in their home repairing antique bisque dolls, which they buy and sell online. These aren't the blessings Charlene had hoped for when she was pregnant with Carla. But they are blessings nonetheless.

19. Suffer Fools Lightly

Those who have prolonged, debilitating illnesses often find that their spouse and friends abandon them. There are many reasons for this, explored in chapter 9. When a spouse or friends turn out to be fools, those with chronic diseases must learn how to suffer fools lightly. Randy John, a chiropractor, pondered this issue. His wife, Susan, has chronic pain from several illnesses. Because of the restrictions imposed by Susan's afflictions, many former friends, including Christian friends, have rejected the couple.

20. Use Your Suffering to Help Others

In chapter 9 you will meet Pat Mierop, whose blindness provides opportunities for her to reach out and counsel younger women who come into her home to help with her diabetes. There is Janine Jacobsen, whose years of living with a colostomy equip her to counsel other women who are about to acquire one. You will also meet Father John Cockayne, a Catholic priest whose cerebral palsy and many other health problems equip him to minister to sick people in his parish.

As I said, I interviewed people for this book who have severe illnesses but manage to remain upbeat, despite their afflictions. I do not mean to imply that everyone with a chronic disease can or should emulate these people. A person with an infirmity might reasonably feel angry if she or he thought I was trying to give advice about how to live better. Each person needs to beat her or his own path through the thicket. My hope is, however, that reading these stories of being sick well can give a glimmer of hope to those who suffer.

Theme Two: The Epidemic

At the risk of redundancy, let me say that this book has two themes. First, a few people have learned how to live rewarding lives despite sickness. Second, there is an increasing epidemic of chronic illness. I will discuss the second theme briefly here and explore it in depth in chapter 4.

The epidemic of chronic illness is largely unrecognized. One of the mysteries this book will address is how such a conspicuous event could be occurring in full public view with so few people talking about it.[18] Many think that our people are getting healthier and healthier. This book will propose a paradox. While we are getting progressively healthier, we are also getting progressively sicker. It depends on your perspective.

Another puzzle I will address is the fact that this problem with chronic diseases saddles women more than men.

The following table shows the percentage of American people who are expected to have at least one chronic disease in future years, according to a study by the RAND Corporation.[19]

This table shows that the number of Americans with chronic illnesses is projected to increase from 133 million in the year 2005 to 171 million in the year 2030. The number of sick people will grow at a faster rate than the number of healthy people. Therefore the percentage of Americans with a chronic condition will increase over the decades, approaching 50 percent by the year 2030.

Since there is a rising tide of chronic illness, we would expect disability rates to be rising also, because some chronic illnesses

Table 1

Percentage of Americans
with a Chronic Illness in Future Years

A Projection

Year	Percent of the Population	Number of Americans with a Chronic Illness
2005	46.2 %	133 million
2010	47.0 %	141 million
2015	47.7 %	149 million
2020	48.3 %	157 million
2025	48.8 %	164 million
2030	49.2 %	171 million

are disabling. Figure 1 shows the trends in disability rates from 1984 through 2002 for children and working-age adults in the United States. Disability rates for these two age groups have been rising, as shown by the upward slope of the two lines. Here *disability* is narrowly defined as the condition of a person requiring personal assistance for at least one of the Activities of Daily Living (ADLs)—eating, getting in/out of bed, getting in/out of chairs, walking, dressing, bathing, and controlling bowels and urination. These upward trends are statistically significant.[20] Although disability rates are declining among the elderly, nevertheless, the trends in disability rates for all ages combined have been increasing in the United States.[21]

There were chronic illnesses in previous centuries. One century ago people lived with tuberculosis as a chronic disease. It was called consumption, because it slowly consumed a person's lungs. Those afflicted were isolated from their families in sanatoriums. Even in biblical times there were chronic illnesses. We read about those who had been disabled for years by blindness, deformities, or paralysis (John 5:1–5). The difference today is the proportion of the population that is afflicted with chronic illnesses, which is much larger than in the past and increasing over time.

There are three reasons for the rapid increase in the number of people with chronic conditions: (1) aging of the population, (2) success of medical science, and (3) increasing obesity.

Figure 1

**Disability Trends 1984–2002 for Working-Age
Adults and Children**

*(The disabled person gets assistance with one
or more Activities of Daily Living.)*

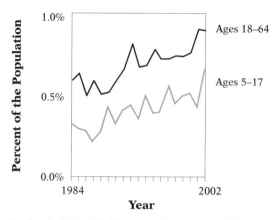

Data from the National Health Interview Survey, courtesy of H. Stephen
Kaye, UCSF Disability Statistics Center

Aging

The primary reason for the rapid increase in the number of people
with chronic conditions is that the risk of acquiring an illness increases with age, and the population is aging. In 1800 the average
lifespan was thirty-six years; in 1900 it was forty-seven years; in 2000
it was seventy-seven years, and soon it will be eighty years.[22] Thus
an increasing proportion of the population acquires a chronic diagnosis, because the average person today is decades older than was
the average person in the past. In previous centuries, if you got sick,
soon you either recovered or died. But today, with our prolonged life
expectancy, we also have prolonged diseases. A person can get sick
and live with the illness for seven decades.

The Success of Medical Science

A second reason for the rising tide of chronic illness is the success of medical science. When we physicians say that we "hope to

cure cancer," what do we mean? We do not necessarily mean that we expect cancer to go away. Rather we mean that we hope to transform cancer from a lethal into a chronic illess.[23] Thus as medicine becomes more powerful in the future, the rates of chronic illnesses will increase because many patients who would otherwise have died will now survive with some chronic diagnosis or other. This will be discussed in chapter 4. When doctors save lives, the patients who are rescued from death are usually those with chronic illnesses, thus a decrease in the death rate usually results in an increase in the rate of chronic illness. In chapter 4 we will see that what is true of cancer is also true of AIDS. We physicians have transformed AIDS from a lethal into a chronic disease.

The hope that future medical breakthroughs (from genetics or stem cell research for example) will solve this problem of chronic illness is deceptive. Medical breakthroughs can be expected to have four impacts on chronic illness: some diseases will be prevented; a few people will be cured; people with chronic illnesses will have a better quality of life; some people who otherwise would have died will live with their chronic diseases. The fourth effect is the way in which future medical breakthroughs will increase the rate of chronic illness.[24]

Many readers have trouble figuring out what I mean when I say that good medical care often increases rather than decreases the amount of chronic illness. Consider my wife Pat. She was in the Intensive Care Unit (ICU) on the brink of death twice a year. If she had not received good medical care, she would have died, which would have decreased by one the number of people living with chronic illness. Because she received good medical care, she survived another six months (until the next medical crisis in the ICU), which increased by six months the amount of time she lived with chronic illness. Excellent medical care saves lives and thereby increases the rate of chronic illness. With poor medical care people with chronic illnesses are more likely to die, which decreases the chronic illness rate but is tragic.

The success of medicine contributes to the increasing rates of chronic illness in another way. We doctors are better at diagnosing these illnesses earlier in the course of the disease than was true in our grandparents' era. The result is that there are more years during which patients are aware of having a chronic illness. This results in an apparent (but not a real) increase in the amount of such illness.

Many of us take medicine for high blood pressure or type 2 diabetes. If our grandparents had these diseases, they lived in blissful ignorance, unaware that they had health problems. Chronic illness looms large in our consciousness, which is a good thing because you have to know it is there before you can control it. In our grandparents' time there was not so much awareness of chronic disease because the diagnostic methods were more primitive. This is part of the "medicalization" of popular culture that has occurred over the past century. We are thinking about our health more than our ancestors did. If we have some defect in our health, we are far more aware of it than they would have been.

Worsening Obesity

The third cause of the epidemic is the obesity that is sweeping the globe. The CDC says that obesity will soon surpass smoking cigarettes as the number one preventable cause of morbidity and mortality.

> [Obesity] is the world's biggest public health issue today—the main cause of heart disease . . . ; the principal risk factor in diabetes; heavily implicated in cancer and other diseases. Since the World Health Organization labeled obesity an 'epidemic' in 2000, reports on its fearful consequences have come thick and fast.
>
> When the world was a simpler place, the rich were fat, the poor were thin, and right-thinking people worried about how to feed the hungry. Now, in much of the world, the rich are thin, the poor are fat, and right-thinking people are worrying about obesity.[25]

Obesity leads to a hornet's nest of other problems, starting with something called the *metabolic syndrome*, which is defined as an increase in abdominal girth, bad cholesterol, high blood pressure and blood sugar.[26] In time this syndrome leads to heart attacks, strokes, diabetes, some cancers, sexual dysfunction, infertility, abnormal menses, polycystic ovaries, gallstones, and increased mortality. Furthermore the weight has destructive effects on the joints, causing increasing arthritis pain from wear and tear on the knees, hips, and spine. Obesity worsens breathing problems, anxiety, and depression. These topics will be explored in depth in chapter 4.

This list helps us understand why more women than men have chronic diseases. On average, women live six years longer than men, therefore they live longer with their medical problems. Furthermore, women are more apt than men to go to a doctor when they have symptoms. Consequently they are diagnosed earlier as having a chronic condition. This leads to better management of the problem, which further contributes to prolonged life expectancy for women. When you add these factors together, you find women living with a diagnosis for more years than men live with a diagnosis. Men are more likely to have no diagnosis (because of avoiding doctors) until late in their disease and to die sooner than women.

Thus the task of figuring out how to have an acceptable lifestyle despite a chronic condition is a puzzle that will interest women more than men. Women are also twice as likely as men to be the unpaid caregivers tending to the needs of chronically sick people (see chapter 8).

In summary, to prevent the increasing epidemic of long-term illnesses, we need to lose weight, stop smoking cigarettes, exercise, and take other health-preserving measures. For those who are afflicted with chronic illness, it is essential to learn how to have fulfilling lives while suffering with such diseases. Since the Baby Boom generation will enjoy a longevity that far surpasses that of their grandparents, they had better learn how to live with health defects without feeling that their lives have been ruined.

About the Author

Before I go on, let me tell you something about myself and my experiences, so you will know who is giving you the information that follows.

I was raised as an atheist and mathematician. During my senior year at Brown University, as I listened to Handel's *Messiah*, I was converted to Christianity. I then got a master's degree in theology at Harvard University and was ordained a minister. I served in a church north of Boston, in Beverly Farms. As I worked with people, I grew interested in chronic illness. I went through medical school, then did a residency in psychiatry at the Yale University School of

Medicine. Because the growth of chronic illness is an epidemic, I studied epidemiology and got a master of public health degree. Then I served on the faculty of the National Institutes of Health (NIH) for seven years, in charge of epidemiologic research on stress and chronic mental disorders.

From the beginning of my psychiatry training, I was motivated by Jesus's value system. In Matthew 25:31–46 he speaks of the last judgment when he will separate the sheep from the goats. He says to the sheep, "Come, you who are blessed by my Father, inherit the Kingdom prepared for you from the foundation of the world. For I was hungry, and you fed me. I was thirsty, and you gave me a drink. I was a stranger, and you invited me into your home. I was naked, and you gave me clothing. I was sick, and you cared for me. I was in prison, and you visited me" (vv. 34–36 NLT).

Puzzled, his listeners ask Jesus what he is talking about. Jesus replies, "I assure you, when you did it to one of the least of these my brothers and sisters, you were doing it to me!" (v. 40 NLT).

I began to realize that people with chronic illnesses were among those whom Jesus refers to as "the least of these my brothers and sisters." From the first day of my psychiatry residency at Yale Medical School, I took an intense interest in the chronically mentally ill—though most other psychiatry residents had no interest in them. My focus has persisted over the last quarter of a century. Today, as chairman of Behavioral Health at Waterbury Hospital (a teaching hospital affiliated with Yale Medical School), I spend half of my time taking care of people with severe and prolonged mental illness, for whom a cure is not an available option. Their diseases have impoverished most of them. Many have lost their family and friends. Many live in a homeless shelter. We are able to help some find apartments to live in.

One man I treat lives in a cave beneath the railroad tracks near the center of the city, even in the wintertime. He is too paranoid to live elsewhere. I wonder sometimes if perhaps he is the one Jesus refers to as "the least of these my brothers and sisters." This man tells me that he lives like a king. The food he harvests from dumpsters is better than the food eaten by royalty, he says. He adores living the way he does, despite the snowstorms. When I talk with him, he makes no sense whatsoever. He has many peculiar ideas that don't go away, even with medication. Though he is paranoid, he is a meek and quiet man, disturbing no one.

My research at the NIH informs the present book. For example, we have observed that social supports—friends and family—turn out to have more impact on how a person copes than does his or her stress. If a person is stricken with a disease, his or her level of distress will vary enormously depending on whether the person is isolated (no friends) or has a social network. When you read Sue Sowle's story in chapter 1, you will see this reflected in her life.

For some time I had been seeking to understand human resilience through medical research and research on the Bible, when it dawned on me that I should turn to the experts. The real experts on chronic illness are those who are afflicted and their unpaid caregivers.

I decided that I wanted to talk to those who remained upbeat despite severe and prolonged illness. I started asking other doctors, clergy, nurses, and friends to refer me to such people. As it became widely known that I was interested in this subject, people began coming out of the woodwork, wanting to tell me their stories. Throughout this research project I have tried to remain open to the Holy Spirit's leading as people with chronic illness just seemed to pop up in my life, as if by miracle. Father John Cockayne is an example of one who found me. One day his voice was on my phone mail, a wobbly voice that was hard to understand because bronchitis and cerebral palsy sapped its full strength. You will read about him in chapter 9.

From the viewpoint of the people I interviewed, this book was a godsend, offering them an unprecedented opportunity to share their wisdom with others. These are mostly quiet people who live obscure lives, the kind of people you would never hear about otherwise, because they don't cross your path. From the viewpoint of my interviewees, it was like receiving a Nobel Prize—public recognition for what they have accomplished.

This book is about the triumph of the human spirit and the Holy Spirit, about heroism and bravery on the battlefield of health. People often don't know what kind of stuff they are made of until they are tossed into the furnace of affliction and melted down, so that the pure gold separates from the dross. Isaiah 48:10 says, "See, I have refined you, though not as silver; I have tested you in the furnace of affliction."

1

How to Survive

In this chapter I use case histories to discuss the first three strategies that help people endure chronic affliction. They are:

1. Cultivate your social network.
2. Keep your priorities straight.
3. Don't dwell on your illness.

First, by way of introduction, let me tell you about a cardiologist,
whom I will call Arvind Patel, respecting his request for anonymity.
Arvind Patel was born in Punjab, India. He immigrated to the United
States at age twenty-four and is a practicing Hindu. He and his wife
worship in a Hindu temple in their city. (Hinduism is the fifth major
religion in the United States, after Christianity, Judaism, Islam, and
Buddhism in that order.)

For the past twelve years Dr. Patel has been living with metastatic
cancer. When he was first diagnosed at age thirty-eight, he was thought
to have a life expectancy of six months. The cancer originated just
below his stomach. It metastasized to his liver. Arvind has had many
operations and radiation. Usually he has discomfort, a sensation that
is not quite strong enough to call pain. He's been taking the medi-

cine interferon daily for a decade. Interferon produces flulike side effects, which Arvind has endured during most of this time—fever, joint aches, muscle aches, and fatigue—and there have been many complications of the cancer, which I won't discuss.

Despite the cancer, Arvind is quietly exuberant about life. This is possible because he does three things. *First,* he has cultivated his social network (strategy one). He has an adoring wife who sticks with him through thick and thin. As a skilled internist, his wife has been the quarterback in charge of Arvind's treatment team. Other members of his social network—his children, family, friends, and professional colleagues—have rallied around him during the crisis points of this disease. Arvind used to love to play tennis. When that became impossible, he took up the card game bridge, which allowed him to interact with others.

Second, Arvind keeps his priorities straight (strategy two). The needs of patients are his highest priority. His patients help him a lot. For example, if a man is having a heart attack at 3 A.M., with crushing chest pain, Arvind will perform an angiogram, including angioplasty and placement of a stent. As a result, the patient feels better and is profoundly grateful. "This experience gives me the biggest high," says Arvind. "It makes me feel great!"

Third, Arvind doesn't dwell on his disease (strategy three). Even when he is uncomfortable, he doesn't ruminate about the cancer nor its prognosis. He works full time as a cardiologist. Work is a blessing, allowing him to forget the discomfort and focus instead on the needs of his patients. A metastasis to his spine caused considerable pain, and a doctor at Sloan Kettering proposed to put Arvind permanently on narcotics. Arvind refused, saying, "Would you want to undergo cardiac catheterization knowing your doctor was taking narcotics?" Instead a neurosurgeon removed the metastasis and local radiation eliminated the pain without narcotics.

Someone who hasn't seen Arvind in years will say, "Why, you look fabulous!" This annoys him. The unstated expectation is that Arvind would have deteriorated because of the cancer. He doesn't want to be identified as a man with cancer. He wants to be known for who he is, an accomplished cardiologist. He has to remind himself that people who say, "You look fabulous," are well meaning even though their comments are stupid. When you meet Arvind, you don't meet "a case of cancer," because Arvind doesn't dwell on his disease, nor does he identify himself with it.

In summary, Arvind lives with uncertainty about his future. He has been able to cope, even though he knows that someday the disease could get worse and he might have to stop working. For a decade he has had flu symptoms, discomfort, and occasional pain. There have been multiple surgeries and complications, but he doesn't allow what he considers minor problems to ruin his life. For him being alive is delicious, and with the coping strategies he is able to find pleasure in life.

Strategy One: Cultivate Your Social Network

When I set up the Crisis Service at Waterbury Hospital fifteen years ago, Sue Reilly worked for me. Since then she has married Steve Sowle, moved to Evanston, Illinois, and earned a master of social work (MSW) degree. They have two children, Andrew and Zachary, and the younger child, Zachary, has multiple birth defects.

I asked Sue if, given a choice, she would sign up to go through again what she has gone through with Zachary.

"In a heartbeat," she replied.

Zachary's birth defects go by the name CHARGE syndrome. CHARGE is an acronym for:

Coloboma (a defect in the iris and retina)
Heart defects
Atresia (absence) of some of the nasal passages
Retardation of development
Genital anomalies
Ear anomalies

Zach, at four and one-half years old, is only now being toilet trained. He is weaker than other kids, and it's still unclear what his cognitive ability will be. For example, his parents don't know if he will be able to go to college or even work at a McDonald's flipping hamburgers. After many operations, his clubfeet have been repaired. During most of his life, Zach has had fifteen different doctors specializing in the care of each of his many problems. Although Zach now eats solid food, for the first four years of his life, he had zero interest in food. People with CHARGE syndrome often have trouble eating, but most of them do eventually learn to eat by mouth. The fact that Zach has started eating is one of the reasons that his geneticist believes Zach has CHARGE syndrome.

Although her husband, Steve, is a born optimist, Sue is not. Her natural disposition tends to be cynical and pessimistic. Thus it is surprising to hear her say she'd go through what she's endured all over again. Her upbeat attitude cannot be attributed to faith. She and Steve are dyed-in-the-wool atheists.

"Our view is that this stuff happens," Sue says, "and we simply have to blunder through it. Actually, I think it is easier to be an atheist when a child is born with defects. We don't ask ourselves why God did this or why God let this happen. We simply accept it as meaningless. That allows us to avoid struggling with the meaning so we can focus on the practical problem of living in the present with Zach's daily challenges.

"Lots of people said they were praying for us," Sue continues. "That was nice, I guess. When people would say to us, 'Everything happens for a reason,' I would wonder, *Exactly what kind of reason could there possibly be for Zach's birth defects?* My view is that CHARGE syndrome probably occurs because of a chromosome deletion that takes place at random."

Sue hasn't always felt positive about their situation. At first, Zach's condition appeared to be a disaster. Sue cried through the entire first year of his life. She often wondered if she were capable of being the mother of a child with so many problems.

Only slowly did the blessings become evident. Over the last five years, all six of Sue's siblings have flown in to spend time with her. Previously she would have said that her family of origin was pleasant but distant. Now she has a warm and intimate relationship with all her brothers and sisters. They have become Sue's safety net.

Zach brought other blessings. Steve was on the faculty of the Chicago Kent College of Law. He had to drop out of the tenure track to have time for the crises at home. He now is assistant dean and teaches at the same college, no longer under pressure to publish.

The assistant dean role fits him better than the tenure track. Had it not been for Zach, Steve would never have discovered his true calling.

Zachary is gregarious. Recently he walked into a waiting room full of strangers, walked up to a woman he didn't know, and asked, "What did you have for lunch today?" He then engaged her in a twenty-minute conversation. He is eager to please, a happy child.

Some of the reason Zach is so popular is that nearly everyone has known him for years in the circles he travels, which is usually the waiting rooms of doctors' offices. People remember this child who was so often in a cast and had a feeding tube up his nose. They are delighted to see that he is now doing better. By *people* I mean adults. Zach has spent his life relating to adults—physical, speech, occupational, and cognitive therapists; doctors; nurses; and medical technicians. With one exception, he doesn't interact with other kids. The exception is Andrew, his older brother, whom Zachary adores and with whom he shares a room. There is laughter coming down the stairs when the two of them are upstairs together.

Ironically, some of the struggle of the first year for Sue arose because Zach was so loveable. Originally his parents expected him to die. They were afraid to allow themselves to fall in love with him. There was a question of leukemia, but it turned out to be nothing. Eventually Sue and Steve let down their guard and were charmed by Zach's magnetic personality.

Things have improved so much for Zach that initially Sue told me that she would be fraudulent if she were interviewed for my book, because, "Zach is fine. He has recovered and everything is fine now. He's just a normal kid."

Can There Be a Reason?

Sue would sign up to go through it all again "in a heartbeat," because this incredible four-and-a-half-year experience has been "a lovely one," she writes in an email. The decisive issue was that Sue discovered a safety net of people who supported her—husband, brothers, sisters, and mother-in-law. When she first learned that her infant had problems, she did not anticipate that the experience could be so rewarding.

Many sick people and their caregivers in this book are cheerful because family and friends support them. A social support network is of vital importance in dealing with stress. It is so powerful that those who are sick but have friends may not even feel stressed, as I said in the introduction.

I want to comment on something Sue said: "When people would say to us, 'Everything happens for a reason,' I would wonder, *Exactly what kind of reason could there possibly be for Zach's birth defects?*" Should we view Zachary's birth defects as meaningless, a development that has no reason? For me that view is difficult to reconcile with the Bible. Jesus says God micromanages the universe so that not a sparrow dies without God's permission and even the hairs on our head are numbered (Matt. 10:29–30; Luke 12:6–7). How then can we understand evil, such as CHARGE syndrome?

The best answer comes from Augustine of Hippo, who explains the existence of evil as follows: "God judged it better to bring good out of evil than not to permit any evil to exist."[1] The reason for an illness is often something that lies in the future, rather than something that lies in the past, as we will discuss in chapter 5.

The Importance of the Safety Net

I asked Sue what it would have been like for her if she had not had a network of people to support her. "Oh God," she replied, "that's just a terrible and frightening thought. It would have been hell! Steve and his mom just took over and raised my older son, Andrew, who was six when Zach was born. Steve's mother was here all the time. She was wonderful! There was a constant stream of people coming to visit us and phone calls every night. It made all the difference. This was not a solo thing. Because of the people around me, I could cry and complain and go back to the hospital again.

"For example," Sue continued, "when Zach was five days old, a decision was made to move him from the local hospital to the Children's Hospital, because he was doing poorly. I came home for dinner before going with him to the Children's Hospital. I needed to grab a handful of things, pack a bag. We sat down for dinner, and I just started to cry uncontrollably. I cried for a full hour. Andrew and Steve just held me and hugged me for that hour. 'Mom needs help,' Andrew said. They were just there for me. At the end of an hour I was strong enough to get up from the dinner table, pack, and leave."

"Have you ever been to a circus and seen the trapeze artists with a safety net under them in case they fall?" I asked.

"Yes!" Sue replied. "Yes, that is exactly it!"

Sue used the first of the twenty strategies—cultivate your social network—that I gave in the introduction, the strategies people use to live well despite chronic illness.

Strategy Two: Keep Your Priorities Straight

Suzanne Luchs, of Milford, Connecticut, and a new member of my church, has lived with pain for many years from fibromyalgia, migraines, and endometriosis. To understand Suzanne's decision to remain upbeat, you have to start with Suzanne as a mother.

Throughout her life she has loved children, any and all children. There was nothing she wanted more in life than to be a mother. So when she got married at age twenty-four, it came as a jolt to discover that she couldn't get pregnant. The decade before her marriage, she had had premenstrual and menstrual pain. Like many women Suzanne had been counseled to ignore these pains. In retrospect, that was bad advice. The pain was evidence of undiagnosed endometriosis, which scarred her fallopian tubes, leading to infertility. The problem could not be fixed despite several surgeries.

In her effort to get pregnant, Suzanne underwent every possible procedure short of retrieving her eggs, fertilizing them in vitro, and implanting the embryos in her uterus. That procedure bothered her ethically. She worried, "What happens to the embryos that are not implanted?"

"There's nothing I ever wanted more than to be a mother," Suzanne says. "By age thirty-seven I was getting the panicky feeling that it would never happen."

Since all else had failed, Suzanne began to explore adoption. Kurt, her husband, was open to, but not enthusiastic about, the idea. Suzanne heard of someone who adopted a child from Romania. "What about Romania?" she asked Kurt.

"No, not right now," he had replied. Kurt vetoed adoption of children from a variety of countries. It turned out that he had the face of an Asian baby in his imagination when he thought of an adopted baby, and the mismatch between his imagination and Suzanne's proposal that they adopt was, with one exception, the source of his veto.

The exception was that one day Suzanne asked, "What about China?"

On that day Kurt envisioned an Asian baby and it seemed right. So he said yes. Many babies are put up for adoption in China each year. Suzanne applied to adopt one. Eventually she and Kurt became the parents of Nora, who is six years old as I write.

As the time came to fly to China to get Nora, Suzanne figured she had to whip herself into better physical shape. She had been physically inactive but was about to begin carrying a nineteen-pound, one-year-old infant. So she decided she needed a crash course at a gym. Without consulting anyone, Suzanne began lifting weights and doing aerobic exercises ninety minutes a day, five days a week.

Her body rebelled. She would drive home from the gym trembling. There was overwhelming exhaustion to the point that she feared falling asleep at the wheel. All sorts of bizarre sensations arose inside her body. She had numbness at the tips of her fingers, burning muscles, constant panic attacks, and weird emotional alarms. When she touched her muscles, they would shake out of control. Her skin began to tingle. She had shooting pains from her back and shoulders, down her arms. When she walked across the room, she felt that her feet might shatter, as if they were brittle, made of fragile ceramic. She had to urinate twenty times a night. She seemed to be disintegrating.

The doctors thought she must have multiple sclerosis (MS). Suzanne imagined her ability to be a mother going down the drain along with her health, destroyed by a progressive, wasting disease. Despair set it, which made the panic attacks worse. An MRI scan of her brain was the first piece of good news. It showed none of the white spots that one would expect from MS. Thus the diagnosis of this mysterious disease became more obscure, except to say that it probably was not MS.

Eventually it became clear that Suzanne had suffered an abrupt onset of fibromyalgia. The diagnosis simply put a name to that mysterious conundrum of problems Suzanne was experiencing. Fibromyalgia itself was a mystery, but the diagnosis meant that she did not have a progressive deteriorating condition like MS. Ironically the term *fibromyalgia* was good news to her, even though her symptoms continued to plague her.

Much of the time Suzanne felt as if her body were on fire, burning from the inside out. She couldn't get away from it. Unless she was distracted, she was tortured. This grew worse when she tried to sleep. On top of it all, she suffered migraine headaches. Once she had a migraine that lasted continuously for one year, despite all kinds of medications at high doses.

You might incorrectly expect that Suzanne would be crushed and bitter because of these afflictions. But you have to remember that she wanted to be a mother above all else. The fact that she did not have a progressive deteriorating condition was good news, because it meant that she could fly with Kurt to China to adopt Nora. Thus, despite her experience of fibromyalgia and migraine pain, she celebrated with relief, because she was able to become a mother. Motherhood trumped pain. It was a question of priorities. For Suzanne pain was present but less important.

"My experience," she says, "is that God is incredibly generous and good! I know this must sound silly, like Pollyanna. I was in extreme physical pain. Whereas the original Pollyanna was blindly and foolishly optimistic, I was optimistic for a reason, namely that I was going to be granted my deepest desire, namely a child. Five years later Kurt and I returned to China and came back with Jia."

Years after the onset of fibromyalgia, Suzanne found Dr. Russell Jaffe, who had a lab to test for delayed allergic reactions.[2] Such allergic reactions would not be found by a normal lab because they are not immediate. In Suzanne's case, they came three days later. Tests showed that Suzanne had a delayed allergic reaction to wheat and gluten. When she stopped eating wheat and gluten, there was an 80 percent reduction in her migraines and fibromyalgia pain.

Suzanne's story demonstrates that suffering can be accepted providing it does not encroach on a person's top priority. Many sick people find that they need to ponder their priorities carefully and decide what is most important. One woman clung to life until her son graduated. Then she relaxed her grip on life and died. Once again, it was a matter of priorities.

For many people children are the top priority. For others it is God. When my wife Pat was alive and we had so many losses, I found Jesus's teachings helpful. Jesus said the top priority should be to love the Lord with all your heart, soul, and strength; and the second priority was to love your neighbor as yourself (Matt. 22:37–39; Mark 12:30–31; Luke 10:27). For many people, their nearest "neighbor" is their child.

Nurturing children and loving God are concerns that are especially helpful to sick people, because no illness can destroy a person's ability to focus on these priorities. Sickness might erode your finances, ruin your physique, end your sex life, and leave your career in shambles, but it cannot destroy your ability to love God, relate to your neighbor, and nurture your child. Keeping these priorities clearly in mind cultivates optimism, because the disease is not able to undermine your top priorities.

Strategy Three: Don't Dwell on Your Illness

The central image for this next case history is a brown paper bag. Perhaps it was used to bring apples or potatoes home from the supermarket. Someday a child may use it to make a mask, after he or she cuts holes for eyes and draws a nose and a mouth. But right now the bag is filled with air, nothing else. You might think that there is little of significance inside an empty brown paper bag, but you would be wrong.

The most jovial, good-natured physician I ever met is Sandy Hamill. His given name is Chalmers but everyone calls him Sandy. When I told him I was writing this book, he said, "I know who you should talk to, Mary ____." (At her request, I'm omitting her last name. That's because she is a member of Alcoholics Anonymous. The idea of using last names doesn't sit well with her.) "Despite terrible arthritis Mary has remained upbeat," Sandy told me, "and brought sunshine into the lives of everyone around her, including me." Sandy smiled, then gave one of his infectious chuckles.

I interviewed Mary at her home in Cheshire, Connecticut, when she was seventy-two years old. She was lying in bed on the first floor of her home, in what had once been a dining room. Mary was delighted to see me. Her family told me she had brightened up for days in anticipation of my visit. Evidently the idea of someone writing a book about "being sick well" appealed to her. It was not every day that a writer proposed that Mary's life was a success and should be recorded to inspire other people. She figured she was an expert on joyful living despite chronic illness.

Mary's hands are conspicuous—the first thing I notice. Her wrists are deformed and her fingers have a sideways S shape that contradicts my knowledge of anatomy. They are pink and soft when I shake them, but feel odd, like a floppy bag of skin with some disconnected bones tossed inside at random. They look useless, like the front fins of an ichthyosaur that might be helpful in the water but limp on land.

I was astonished to hear that Mary still wrote all the checks and kept the checkbook for the family. Two decades earlier, when her arthritis got so bad that she could no longer turn the keys to start her car, she took a fork from the kitchen, and inserted it through the middle of the key ring. That gave her a handle she could use to leverage the keys to start the car. When I interviewed her, Mary still drove, even though she could not grasp the wheel because her fingers wouldn't wrap around it. The car had fine-tuned power steering, so it turned with even the slightest pressure from the palm of her hand on the wheel, so she was able to drive safely.

Mary couldn't understand why I was so impressed with her hands. She had lived with these hands for decades and now took them to be "normal." It is astounding what people accept as normal!

Over the years, as her joints failed from rheumatoid arthritis, Dr. Richard Matza replaced many of the joints in her fingers, wrists, toes, ankles, and knees. There was a waxing and waning pain that was a permanent part of Mary's life. I couldn't get her to talk about the pain. She shrugged it off and changed the subject. I found an old newspaper report, which said that, prior to her surgeries, Mary had been in so much pain that she needed to use her teeth to pull the sheet up over her in bed.

Her sister, Rose Bradley, told me that Mary's pain once got so bad that she went to a hospital in Boston to have specialized surgery to replace the joint where her jaw hinged on her skull (the TMJ joint). But on admission to the hospital a chest X-ray detected a small lung cancer. Instead of jaw surgery, she had a lobe of her lung removed. That cured the cancer. She never did get her jaw joint replaced.

If this woman, who talks so much, has jaw pain, you could have fooled me. She shows no evidence of it. All I can see as I watch her jawbone is a love of conversation, an addiction to dialogue, and a deep-seated interest in people. She wants to know all about my children and me.

Mary's outlook on life is always cheerful. She starts the conversation by clarifying that her natural tendency to look on the bright side of life is a personality characteristic that she was born with. "It's chemical," she says. "I simply am that way because of my chemistry. I think your readers should know that I don't choose to be happy. It is simply my personality. And faith. It comes from my faith in God."

Mary was brought up Catholic but hasn't gone to church in years. She prays at home. No clergy, other than me, have visited her.

Three decades earlier, when she worked as a real estate agent, Mary got so crippled that she could no longer go into houses with her clients. She knew almost all the houses in Cheshire. Over the years she had sold many of them more than once and knew exactly what they looked like on the inside. So she would advise her clients what to look for, then send them in on their own while she waited in the car.

When Mary's arthritis became more severe and she became disabled, she refused to sit around and do nothing. She took up duplicate bridge, a competitive form of the card game. That took her to Canada and Atlanta for tournaments. Since she could no longer play golf, Mary was determined to play some sport, and competition bridge was her new passion. It was during Mary's bridge playing years that she got into heavy drinking. She went into rehab, then became a committed AA member.

Mary's other hobby is reading books. She devours both fiction and nonfiction.

"Mary is the smartest of the bunch of us," her sister Rose, who is a nun, tells me. "Mary has always been a go-getter. My brother has a Ph.D., but I always say that Mary has two Ph.D.s because of all the books she reads and how many things she is interested in.

"Mary stays in that bedroom a lot," Rose continues. "But she is always thinking about other people. She has large phone bills. She is constantly in touch with our family members and has a couple of women from AA for whom she is a sponsor and mentor.

"She refuses to talk about her disease," Rose says. "She will not tell you if she is in pain. When she has a bad day she doesn't phone anyone that day. She waits until she feels better before being in contact. At one family gathering she got a brown paper bag and said that anyone who mentioned anything about disease would have to put five dollars in the bag. With the threat of losing five bucks, everyone avoided talking about her illness. The conversation was about the exciting things that we were doing, about Peter and Meg, Mary's grandchildren, and about the exhilarating side of life. Mary loves that kind of talk. She thrives on it."

Mary's parents came to the United States in 1928. Her father, who was English, was a conscientious and moral man. He came first and found a job so he was able to support a wife before he went back two years later to fetch his Irish sweetheart. They settled in Nahant, a peninsula in the ocean in Lynn, north of Boston. Together they had five children, of whom Mary is the oldest. Her dad worked hard to support the family and was a nurturing parent.

"Mary takes after our father," says Rose. "She has his personality."

When you meet Mary, you do not meet a woman crushed by rheumatoid arthritis. If she hadn't talked about pain medicine with Elba Armstrong, a visiting nurse who popped in, I would never have known Mary was currently in pain. What eclipses the pain and disability is her delightful personality, apparently the chemistry she inherited or learned from her father. It just comes naturally to her, like water running downhill.

As I said good-bye to the family, Mary insisted that I take with me a poinsettia that was so huge I could barely see around the red petals to find my way out the front door. It was five days before Christmas.

Driving home, I thought about how often I have given advice to patients who suffer from chronic pain. "Eventually you have to make a decision," I tell my patients. "You have to decide what is going to be the focus of your life. If you talk all the time about your pain, then at first your friends will be sympathetic. But after a few months they won't know what to say. It becomes very old. Your friends may even avoid you, because they feel helpless and don't know what to do or say to help you. Many people with chronic pain have consciously decided not to talk about it, because the pain should not be the central issue in life. If all your conversations revolve around your suffering, then all your thoughts will revolve around it also. There are more important things in life. You don't want to miss out on the fullness of life simply because of pain."

That is solid advice. But few heed it. "I can't enjoy life until someone first gets rid of this pain," they tell me. I was delighted to meet Mary, because she lives happily by the counsel I've given to others.

Today other problems are looming for Mary. At age seventy-two she and her husband are considering selling their house and moving to an assisted-living facility. Even if she had never had arthritis, the problems of old age would now be on her agenda.

Epilogue

About two weeks after my second visit to Mary's home, she died. This took me by surprise. She had painful leg ulcers that she refused to talk about, but they were getting progressively worse. They proved fatal.

This reminded me of another woman named Elise Christianson, who went to my church. I interviewed Elise about her cancer. She minimized the whole thing and wanted to talk about serving the needs of others. Overall I found Elise so upbeat that she hoodwinked me into believing she didn't have much of a problem. It was manageable, not a burden. I decided not to include Elise in my book because I believed she wasn't dealing with a severe illness. Cancer was a relatively unimportant part of her life. I was astounded when she died two weeks later.

In the cases of both Elise and Mary I had failed to recognize the gravity of their illnesses because they didn't want to talk to me about their problems. In both cases it was only after they died that it dawned on me that they had been dealing with extreme situations. This illustrates a phenomenon I'll discuss at the end of this book: Sometimes people who have severe diseases or who are caring for someone with a severe chronic condition may appear to carry a light burden. Sue Sowle, who no longer considers herself burdened by Zach's many birth defects, is an example of this.

Mary's daughter, Carol Johnstone, told me that I had given Mary a great gift by listening to and writing down her story. Much of what I wrote was read at Mary's funeral.

As Normal as Possible

A patient of mine who has half a dozen chronic diseases and takes a dozen medicines, taught me a simple wisdom. "I get great pleasure out of going over to help with my grandchildren," she said. "I love seeing those little faces light up. It's surprising the things those kids say. The main thing is not to dwell on my troubles. I've got to live as normal a life as I can, accomplish as much as I can."

My mother is ninety years old and lives in an assisted-living facility near me. Every day she eats one meal in the common dining room with her friends. She says that her friends have all agreed on one ironclad rule to make meals pleasant: no discussion of medical problems at the dinner table. They are following the third strategy: Don't dwell on your illness.

Returning to the brown paper bag, Mary set it out prominently at a party and said that anyone who mentioned her illness would have to put five dollars in the bag. The emptiness of the bag at the end of the party signifies that the party was a success because Mary's disease was not discussed that evening.

It's interesting that the vast majority of the people I've interviewed for this book were happy to have me use their real names. They've all signed consent forms. They all want others to know that life is worth living, even with a chronic illness, but if we dwell on our problems, we'll be letting life pass us by.

2

A SURVIVOR'S ATTITUDE

The concept of Quad Rugby is at first astonishing, because *quad* refers to "quadriplegic"—someone with a neck injury to the spinal cord leaving him or her paralyzed in all four limbs. Rugby, of course, is the British form of football, played with a ball that is a hybrid between a soccer ball and a pregnant American football. Rugby players are famous for being tough and mean, which this bumper sticker makes clear: "Give blood, play rugby!" You might ask, "How in blue blazes can quadriplegics play rugby?"

When this game was first invented in the 1970s in western Canada, it was named Murder Ball due to the aggressive nature of the game. It grew out of ice hockey and wheelchair basketball. Brad Mikkelson, who formed the first United States team, the Wallbangers, changed the name to Quad Rugby in 1981.[1] The sport has spread around the world and is now the fastest growing of all wheelchair sports.

It is a contact sport played in specialized wheelchairs built for speed. They are able to turn on a dime, spin in circles like a figure skater, and make sharp S curves easily. The only source of power is the player's arms and hands. The player wears no crash helmet. There is no blood spilled during the games.

Coach Al Steiger, an able-bodied rugby player, invited me to a practice of the Connecticut Jammers Quad Rugby Club. He told me something intriguing that took me a while to figure out. He said that he played on an able-bodied rugby team (the Connecticut Grey Rugby Football Club) and coached the Jammers Quad Rugby team. Last year the two clubs played a rugby match, and the able-bodied team had been thoroughly beaten. "They had their butts kicked," was the exact phrase Al used.

I could not imagine how that was possible. It boggled my mind. Rugby players are known to be rugged and ruthless. As good as a team might be in wheelchairs, even allowing for the wheelchairs inflicting some severe bruises on the ankles of the able-bodied men running around on the grass, I would expect that a normal rugby team could run circles around and even leap over the wheelchairs and throw or kick the rugby ball seventy-five yards down the field. I could not imagine how a team of quadriplegics could defeat a fully trained rugby team playing with all its strength, no holds barred. It was utterly inconceivable.

But as often as I asked about it, Al insisted it was true. And he said so in a matter-of-fact tone of voice, as if it were nothing unusual, as if no one should be surprised. His tone astounded me more than anything. Clearly Al was not joking.

Strategy Four: Adopt a Positive Attitude

Al gave me directions by email to a practice of the Jammers. The directions were to a gym and not to a grassy field. Up until then I had a picture in my head of Quad Rugby being played on a grassy field, as rugby games in England are played. But when I got the email directions from Al, the fantasies began to disintegrate. The practice was going to be located inside a basketball gym at 7:00 P.M., which meant that there would be no grass and no hundred-yard playing field.

I parked in a deserted parking lot on a cold night in October. There was no difficulty finding my way into the building. As I walked into the gym, I noticed that the atmosphere was euphoric. These players were having the time of their lives! They were ecstatic and greeted me with delight, even though they had no idea who I was. About ten people in wheelchairs were kidding around with one another, careening their wheelchairs backwards and forwards, in and out, bobbing and weaving, squealing rubber on the polished wood floor. They were talking, bantering, joking, giggling, whooping, laughing, and dribbling the ball—which was smaller than a rugby ball, more like a soccer ball—as they sped down the basketball court.

The wheelchairs were unlike anything I had ever seen before, with a twenty-degree camber (tilt) to the wheels so that the wheels were much farther apart at the bottom than at the top. This meant that the wheelchair was extremely stable and the person's elbows were not knocking into the top of the wheel. The wheel spokes were covered with smooth plastic, so no one's fingers could get caught. There were no armrests. The seats were low, so there was a low center of gravity. The player's toes were tucked far in, with Velcro holding the legs in, and there was a bumper for protection in front of the toes for high-speed crashes against other wheelchairs. The small front wheels, part of normal wheelchairs, were absent. This allowed the big wheels to be brought forward under the person's center of gravity. Thus the player's entire weight was carried on only two wheels. There were also many tiny casters at the front and back of the wheelchair, which kept it from tipping over. The chair had no handles, so it could not be pushed by someone else. Since it was built for collisions, like a bumper-car, it was armored with steel plates. Overall, the wheelchairs looked like battle-scarred chariots from the Roman Empire.

I expected the Quad Rugby team to be all men, but I sat down in a wheelchair beside Cynthia Gadow, who looked to be in her thirties. She began flirting with me and was giggling and joking with the other men as well. She introduced me to Ricky Famiglietti in the wheelchair on my other side who had single-handedly, she said, gotten legislation passed last year in Connecticut to allow disabled people to earn up to seventy-five thousand dollars in any job without getting in trouble with Medicaid. I was impressed. Rick smiled modestly, which conveyed to me the impression that it must be true.

This is a team of movers and shakers, I thought.

"Hey Rich," Cynthia yelled to another player, "way to go!" as Rich Hearn's wheelchair zoomed down the gym at about fifteen miles an hour while he dribbled the ball. Quickly I learned that Cynthia, in addition to being a spirited player, was also the morale builder and cheerleader for the team. Everyone loved having her around.

Al Steiger introduced me to the team, then sent them on twenty laps around the perimeter of the gym. Off they went, zooming around like Manhattan taxicabs in rush hour.

When Al blew the whistle, they gathered in a circle in the center of the gym. I stood just outside the circle with my clipboard under my arm. Near me was a gigantic man named Pete, with shaved head. At first I noticed how muscular his arms were, as if he had been lifting weights and was a bodybuilder. Then I noticed his forearms. They were not wasted at all. I had relaxed enough so that I was beginning to think like a doctor. To be classified as a quadriplegic, a person must have a neck injury in the cervical spine, which is called the C section of the spine. The higher the injury the less function one has in the arms and hands and the more atrophy of muscles. Most wheelchair rugby players are those with more mild cord injuries, ranging from the high (severe) end of C5 to the low (mild) end of C7–8. A partial injury to the spinal cord is much less destructive and far preferable, if you were to have a choice, which no one ever does.

Pete's forearms were muscular, with no evidence of atrophy. His hands worked fine. Even more remarkable, his abdominal and back muscles were strong. Most remarkable of all, his leg muscles were powerful. His quads bulged. I could not imagine how Pete could be a quadriplegic. My disorientation grew worse when Pete climbed out of the wheelchair and began walking around, helping Al and appearing quite athletic. Finally, I realized Pete was not a quadriplegic at all. He was a volunteer. In addition to Al, who was the coach, there were four volunteers. Quad Rugby draws volunteers like a magnet attracts iron filings.

Cynthia also climbed out of her wheelchair at one point. She walked awkwardly and with a cane. I could see she would need a wheelchair because she would tire before long. I walked out on the gym floor and stood beside Cynthia to ask her a few questions. That was dangerous. She was fielding balls as rugby players tossed them to her, squealed their wheelchairs in a sharp U-turn behind her, and zoomed out in front of her at fifteen miles an hour while she rolled the ball on the floor like a bowling ball to challenge the player to scoop it up. Every time I had to leap sideways out of the way or risk getting my ankle broken. Cynthia was cheering and shouting encouragement to each player as if each one were her favorite.

I struck up a conversation. Cynthia said she had been in an automobile accident nineteen years ago that had broken her neck, back, and leg. She had partial injuries to her cervical and lumbar spinal cord. The rule in Quad Rugby is that if you have a combination of upper and lower body deficits you may be allowed to play. Seven years ago Cynthia gave birth to twin boys. Now she was going through a divorce. Having heard that much I hurried back to the safety of my own wheelchair at the side of the gym.

When I came to watch the Quad Rugby practice, I expected to see people with high cervical injuries—perhaps C3 or C4—playing. Instead, I saw people who were skilled in the use of their hands and arms, and it took some argument in my head to convince myself that these were quadri- and not para-plegics. Only one of the players, Jeff Johnson—who is called Murf—had any visible atrophy in his forearm. Murf was in a motorcycle accident at age twenty-six, causing a partial spinal cord injury at C6. He was now thirty-one years old.

As I watched the Quad Rugby players spinning around the gym, I thought, *What a triumph of the human spirit that it does not require a totally functional body to enjoy life!* I am sure that most of these people were depressed when they were first paralyzed. But life goes on. People adapt. They learn to live with it. They work around obstacles, even big ones like loss of their spinal cord. I'm sure that at first they rebelled, told God that their paralysis was unacceptable, prayed for healing, wondered why God had been so sadistic and why he had abandoned them, and on and on. But now, just a few years later, here they were having so much enjoyment that they could barely contain themselves. Their laughter was so contagious that it infected me, a complete stranger. Although they were still paralyzed, apparently the burden of illness had lifted.

Al Steiger was an incredible coach. A recreational therapist from Gaylord Hospital, Todd Munn, had recruited Al from the Connecticut Grey Rugby Football Club to coach the Jammers. On the gym floor Al was in command. He knew exactly what every player was doing. He was cool, calm, collected, and he had a plan. Often coaching from a wheelchair, he was also an excellent wheelchair player.

A reality check: I once again asked Al the question. "Say, Al, didn't you say that once a year this team plays against your able-bodied rugby team?"

"Yup, and we kicked their butt because we are so good!"

I was beginning to feel spacey. It made no sense!

Al set the team to another form of practice. He or one of his helpers would roll a rugby ball down the gym at high speed (like a bowling ball) parallel to the wheelchair, which was zipping down the court at a similar speed. The player had to move close to the rolling ball, reach over, and scoop it up. Squeezing the ball between the player's hand and the chair's wheel brought the ball spinning backward, up, and forward along the rim of the wheel. Then suddenly the ball would flip over the top onto the player's lap, which is the usual place to carry a Quad Rugby ball. However, one of the absolute rules is that you must bounce the ball at least once during every high-speed chase down the speedway.

There was another exercise in which two teams were competing with each other. There were parallel rows of orange cones. Each team's player had to snake zigzag through the orange cones, like slalom skiing, bounce the ball at least once, make a U-turn, speed back, and fling the ball thirty feet to the next player in the tag team.

Finally, the high point of the evening was the scrimmage. Al called for a scrimmage earlier than usual because he knew I had to leave and he wanted me to see the real thing.

Scrimmage

Two orange cones at each end of the basketball court mark the goals. The purpose of the game is to wheel your chair between the goal markers with the ball, having bounced the ball at least once. By passing through the cones with the ball you score a point. More often than not you would have bounced it several times and would hold the ball out at arm's length in triumphant glory for everyone to see as you roll across the goal line. If you roll your wheelchair slowly, it demonstrates that you are gloating because you are not being hassled by the other team's players.

The game is fast moving, almost like ice hockey, but with less space between players and more frequent collisions. It is a high contact sport—one collision every ten seconds, but compared to ice hockey, the collisions in Quad Rugby are less violent and there is less danger to life and limb. In ice hockey all the energy of a collision is absorbed into two human bodies, whereas in Quad Rugby the majority of the energy is absorbed into the steel chariot.

The wheels of the chairs can lock together like the horns of two bucks in combat during mating season. Then it takes a combined effort of opposing teammates to extricate the locked chairs. Sometimes, when the ball is being tossed in from the sidelines, all ten wheelchairs would swing in tiny arcs and get locked into a traffic jam near one goal. Then, when it was clear that both teams were frozen in a logjam, suddenly the entire field became fluid again. Everyone was in motion in tiny semicircles and S curves, this way and that, rubber tires squealing.

When the scrimmage is over and I am picking up my clipboard to leave, a light bulb goes on in my head. Aha! It suddenly dawns on me that perhaps when the able-bodied rugby team, the Grey Rugby Football Club, plays against the Jammers, both teams play in wheelchairs! That idea had never occurred to me before. That would explain why the able-bodied team lost. Of course, they would lose! Al must have thought I understood that.

When I ask Al about it, he says, "Of course," as if it were obvious!

And it really was. No able-bodied person could control a Quad Rugby wheelchair and play the game without bumping into a wall.

Two months earlier my son Matthew and I visited a practice session of the Gaylord Quad Tennis Club. The tennis wheelchairs were similar to the rugby wheelchairs, and when I sat in one, I was unable to turn left or right except with great concentration. It also took effort to go forward in a straight line. It was like going straight in a kayak that has no keel because it is built for whitewater. Since a kayak is built to turn on a dime, when you put your paddle in the water on the right, you instantly turn to the left. The wheelchairs worked in a similar way.

The most unnerving problem is the subtlest: balance. Every able-bodied athlete depends on balance. In a Quad Rugby wheelchair your center of gravity is wobbling atop two large wheels, as if you were on a wiggly, narrow beam, with no way to use your arms to keep your balance. The two large wheels are directly under your center of gravity. The casters are always a bit off the floor, so you are teeter-tottering, first forward slightly, then backward just enough to be aware of being unstable, lurching and tilting. Your toes are tucked far in under you. Your legs are strapped in with Velcro. Your hands are occupied handling the wheels. If you were to topple, as players sometimes do, how would you stop yourself from crashing?

Anyone who wants to learn more about Quad Rugby can go to the U.S. Quad Rugby website (www.quadrugby.com). Quad Rugby is part of something called adaptive sports, which means sports adapted to disabilities. The American Therapeutic Recreation Association website (www.atra-tr.org) will help you learn more about such sports, for example, skiing or kayaking for those who have no legs or no control of their legs. The Jammers are part of the Gaylord Sports Association, which is affiliated with Gaylord Hospital near where I live in central Connecticut.

Other Game Plans

As I drove home, worried whether I would get home before the deadline set by our babysitter Nicole, I thought about Jim Lubin, a quadriplegic I had met when surfing the web and with whom I have corresponded by email. Jim has a spinal cord injury at C2, a level so high that he lost total use of his arms, hands, and trunk. It was not an automobile accident but a bizarre disease that struck abruptly in his early twenties. Since he was almost totally paralyzed, when he went to rehabilitation, he was bored because there was nothing he could do.

Jim was permanently dependent on a respirator, which, you might at first think, would be a life of torture. But Jim could control some of the airflow in his mouth, so a device was attached to the air tube that could read the direction of airflow in and out of his throat. This device could translate that information into Morse code and transmit it to a computer. Using such a form of data transfer, Jim was able to control a computer, typing seventeen words a minute. With a computer, he mastered the Internet.

Jim has become one of the most gracious hosts in cyberspace, with an ingenious site that is chockablock full of useful information for those who are disabled. His site is called "disABILITY Information and Resources" (www.makoa.org). *Makoa* is a Hawaiian word that means "courageous." Jim spends nine hours a day on the computer. As a webmaster Jim developed a cybernetics "body." Although he could not play Quad Rugby, in a sense Jim does play Internet rugby.

Still in the fast lane on the highway, I thought about Brooke Ellison, who when in the seventh grade had been hit by a car. This caused a high neck injury, causing quadriplegia similar to Jim's. She became permanently dependent on a respirator, because she could not breathe on her own.

Brooke was a bright girl and wanted to go back to school. Her mother, Jean, took her back to school, and became Brooke's constant companion, raising her own hand when Brooke had a question, turning the pages when Brooke was reading a book. Since Brooke's tongue was the only muscle she could control, a simple keyboard device was attached to the roof of her mouth. Through that keyboard Brooke could control a computer that would also control her electric wheelchair. In May 2000 Brooke graduated magna cum laude from Harvard University, and her story was carried on the front page of the *New York Times*.[2]

These quadriplegics and computers! Amazing! At Gaylord Hospital they told me that someone who cannot control any muscle can still control a computer through brain waves. If the human spirit cannot connect with the body, it can still connect with the world via digital technology.

I was now on the exit ramp, getting closer to home. I thought about when I was ten years old, in the mid-1950s, when positive pressure ventilators (respirators) became widely used. Prior to that time any person who sustained a high neck injury, causing quadriplegia sufficiently severe as to be unable to breathe, would have died. This illustrates how breakthroughs in medicine increase the number of chronically ill (see chapter 4 where I will discuss the "caribou effect").

Thinking about these heroic people kept my mind alert enough so that I could drive safely, and I got home at precisely the time set by Nicole, to the minute.

Epilogue

It has now been three years since I visited the Quad Rugby practice and wrote the essay you just read. Since then, in the annual wheelchair rugby match between the Jammers and the Connecticut Grey Rugby team, the Jammers have won every year.

Contrary to what you might think, the joy of life does not necessarily end when a person gets a chronic disease or becomes disabled. The Quad Rugby players illustrate the fourth strategy: Adopt a positive attitude.

Arthur Kleinman, a psychiatrist who studied how people adapt to chronic illness, wrote, "There are many persons with chronic disorders and even severe disabilities who live lives of exemplary courage and often of remarkable stability and success. . . . It is important [to focus on people] whose adaptation to illness is an undoubted success, whose illness problems are effectively dealt with in personal and medical settings, whose life is a model of mastery and grace under fire."[3]

Strategy Five: Avoid Disaster

The next story illustrates the fifth strategy: Avoid disaster. As I said in the introduction, sick people fear three things above all else: impoverishing their families, losing their independence, and becoming a burden to others. For the chronically ill, life is more joyful if they can avoid these disasters.

Sharon (a pseudonym) was twenty-three when she gave birth to her only child, Tom Jr. Six months later it was time for the baby's DPT and polio vaccinations. But there was a flaw in that particular batch of polio vaccine. It contained live polioviruses.

Without knowing it, the pediatrician gave the infant live poliovirus. The baby was fine and never got sick. The virus passed into the baby's stool and somehow entered the mother, perhaps through a cut in her finger. Sharon was one of the seven people in the United States who contracted polio from that defective batch of vaccine. She suffered excruciating pain. At first, the doctors had no idea what was wrong. Eventually the pain subsided and left her muscles paralyzed from her belly button to her toes. There was a lawsuit and she won some money but not enough, of course, to compensate for her loss.

At Gaylord Rehabilitation Hospital, the therapists taught her how to walk with leg braces, do housework from a wheelchair, and drive a car using hand controls. "My husband was helpful because he kept yelling at me, saying, 'Stop feeling sorry for yourself! You must force yourself to do this. You can do it!' That helped bolster my will power, so that I was able to learn an entirely new lifestyle."

For two years after Sharon got polio, she and her baby lived with either her parents or her in-laws. At first her husband, Tom, lived there also, but during those two years Tom had an affair. He later returned to Sharon. Two years after the polio struck, Sharon and Tom established their own residence. Life was more satisfying when Sharon was not living with either her parents or in-laws, because she disliked being dependent.

"It took two years to get independent of our parents," she says. "Something stuck in my mind. Someone at Gaylord Hospital said, 'You need to get away from all these people. You need to be independent, because they will get tired of having to do things for you. They will feel you are a burden. And that will drive you crazy.'"

Of the three disasters sick people fear, the first was not a problem for Sharon. "Many sick people have financial troubles," she said. "It is a nightmare for them. Fortunately I never did. My husband had good health insurance through his work. He had a wonderful job and made great money, so finances were not a problem. Also at Gaylord they help you apply for Social Security disability."

The second and third disasters were battles for Sharon for two years—losing her independence and becoming a burden to others—but eventually she triumphed over these.

"I got tired of asking people to do things for me," she says. "It weakened my spirit to have to ask my sister to help me get on the toilet or my husband to help me into or out of the bathtub. I had to retrain myself. Even though I couldn't do things the same way I used to, I forced myself to learn other ways to get the job done. They would say, 'Let's see if we can take Sharon to the store,' and that bothered me.

"No one actually did resent me," she continues. "Quite the opposite. If anything, my family was overindulgent. But I said to myself, 'This is ridiculous!' At Gaylord Hospital I had seen people who did nothing but whine all day. That's just not in my personality. I didn't want to give up parenting my son. I'm just willful like that. Being strong-willed helped me gain my independence."

Disability is a tricky concept. In part it is determined by a person's degree of impairment, but only in part. It is also determined by the attitude of other people and the extent to which the environment presents barriers, such as curbs or stairs. To a large extent a person's level of disability is determined by the person's own attitude. I have known many healthy people who are crippled by their attitude, and I have known a quadriplegic on a respirator who tells me he doesn't think of himself as disabled.

"Today I don't have a disability," Sharon says, twenty-seven years after getting polio. "This has become my way of life. It takes me longer to do things because of the paralysis, but I have a rich and rewarding life. People come to me with their problems. I've always been a good listener, so that makes me feel good, being able to help others."

I asked her what was the hardest part of learning to be independent in the first two years after she got polio.

"Of all the things I had to adjust to, the most frustrating was getting my leg braces on and standing up by myself," Sharon replied. "My husband would put the hardware on my legs before he went to work in the morning. It made me so sad, him having to do all that then going off to a full day's work. I couldn't stand it! So one day I sat on the floor, which was a change because at Gaylord they had me sitting on a mat fourteen inches high. The hardest part of putting on my braces was that the shoes were attached to the braces. So I unlatched the knee so I could bend my knee to tie the shoe on my foot. Then I'd straighten my leg and latch the knee again so it was rigid. Then I rolled over onto my tummy so my feet were in a corner against the wall, with my toes pointing down. I used my hands to crawl backwards so my butt rose up higher and higher in the air. I kept saying to myself, 'You can do this!' Standing up was quite an accomplishment. I grabbed hold of my Loft Strand crutches, and they allowed me to get up to a standing position and get balanced."

Hearing details about how Sharon dealt with braces, crutches, and the toilet makes it sound like all the battles have to do with learning how to do things. But the real battle is for independence, which produces self-respect. Sharon was determined to be independent; she refused to allow herself to be defined as disabled.

"With this kind of disability you get to have strong arms," she continued. "You have to protect your upper body, because it is all you have. Every day it got easier. It got to be a routine. Mostly I was afraid I might fall. At Gaylord there had always been an aide there to help me, and to catch me if I lost my balance. Still, even at Gaylord I had some crashes. They teach you how to fall.

"To clean the house," Sharon continues, "I would draw an imaginary boundary line around every room at thirty-six inches above the floor. First I would clean the top half of each room with my braces on. Then I would take my braces off and clean the bottom half, I mean like vacuuming. I vacuumed from my wheelchair. You have to understand that we live in a split-level home with stairs. It is the worst house design in terms of being wheelchair inaccessible. The washing machine is in the basement! I would put all the clothes into a laundry bag so I could get them to the basement and back upstairs.

"I did my grocery shopping from a wheelchair," she says. "I taught myself how to get in and out of a car with braces.

"You get very fatigued at the end of a day," Sharon continues. "I mean, you really beat yourself up and get exhausted. So I take a nap every afternoon. My husband supports my doing that."

I asked Sharon about the affair that Tom had.

"Ninety-nine percent of disabled women have husbands who have affairs or leave them," she replied.

"What about disabled men?" I asked. "Do their spouses leave them?"

"Probably," said Sharon. "At Gaylord Hospital the physical therapist said to me, 'You'd better get ready, because your husband may stray!' Gaylord prepared me for everything. Those marriage vows, 'To have and to hold, in sickness and in health until death do us part,' are fragile. Tom left me for another woman. We were separated a year and a half. Eventually the other woman gave him an ultimatum. 'I'm moving to Florida,' she said. 'You can either come with me or break up.' Tom had a son here. He couldn't leave. Eventually he came back to me."

"What brought him back?" I asked.

"I don't know," Sharon replied. "Maybe because we have always been best friends. We've been together since the eighth grade. We're devout Catholics. Divorce was not part of our upbringing. He came back, and we've had a wonderful marriage ever since. My paralysis never reduced my sexual pleasure, but I've always said, even if Tom didn't love me, the most important thing is that he remains my best friend.

"This disease didn't just happen to me," says Sharon. "It happened to my husband and my child too. It affected everyone around, our families and friends. Everyone's life changed. Fortunately my family and friends stuck by me. It took me two years to adjust to this polio. I say 'two years' because that is how long it took us to become independent of our parents."

Sharon's story illustrates the fifth strategy: Avoid disaster. For those who are healthy, long-term care insurance is a good investment, because it allows you to avoid these three disasters if and when you need chronic care. People with chronic conditions who have good health insurance tend to be happier than those who don't. Those who move out of nursing homes or reduce the burden they impose on others tend to be happier. There is an independence movement sweeping through America. People with severe disabilities are moving out of institutions or leaving their parents' homes and establishing their own apartments and taking responsibility for parenting their own kids. Even quadriplegics on respirators are successfully doing this.

A Unique Focus

This chapter has been about attitude. There are many inspiring books written by motivational experts and management consultants aimed at helping you solve problems and find a positive approach to life, books like *Who Moved My Cheese?* by Spencer Johnson, *The Purpose-Driven Life* by Rick Warren, *The Power of Positive Thinking* by Norman Vincent Peale, *You Can't Afford the Luxury of a Negative Thought* by Peter McWilliams, *Seven Habits of Highly Effective People* by Stephen Covey, and the Chicken Soup for the Soul series.

With one exception *Being Sick Well* is like those other motivational books. The one exception is that this book focuses on the half of the population that suffers from chronic illness. It is a motivational book for those learning to live with sickness.

3

ALTERNATIVES TO COMPLAINING

More often than not people with serious chronic illnesses are out in the workplace, earning a living, just like people without a chronic condition. When we think of chronic illness, we usually think of someone who is disabled, unable to work. We may not realize that there are people working in our office who are in pain or disabled in some way. Winston Churchill said, "Eighty-five percent of the world's work is done by people who don't feel very well." People who struggle to go to work every day despite a chronic illness often survive by relying on the two strategies presented in this chapter: Use humor and take one day at a time.

Strategy Six: Use Humor

Humor is one of the most powerful strategies that sick people use to contend with the problems associated with illness, problems such as tyrannical insurance companies, overpriced medications, stupid doctors and nurses, or the unspeakable indignities of disease. Humor keeps sick people in touch with friends and lightens the mood surrounding a disease.

Although the first part of this chapter deals with the strategy of using humor, do not expect it to be funny. The wit of sick people is odd and difficult to reproduce. Readers who aren't living with a particular disease are likely to say, "Well, I don't think that's anything to laugh about. In fact this seems kind of 'sick' to me."

This humor is often peculiar and dark, but it has healing properties. It defuses tense situations and allows folks to be more human, offering an invitation: *Look, let's step outside this situation and see how absurd it is.* Because sickness is so grim, others often treat sick people grimly. Laughter can turn the grim to a grimace and then into real glee. Often humor rescues human sympathy and respect from the jaws of tragedy.

Humor is idiosyncratic, so I will give you several examples to illustrate different styles. Perhaps one of them will appeal to your sense of what is funny.

Emails of Bette Furn

Bette Furn is a Ph.D. psychologist who practices in Woodbury, Connecticut. She writes emails to her closest friends about her experiences with breast cancer treatment over the course of four years. I will translate Bette's cryptic email style into plain English without changing Bette's content. Although some of Bette's ridicule is directed at people at Yale Medical School, Bette continues going to Yale because she is so impressed with Dr. Barbara Burtness, a leading expert in breast cancer treatment.

SEPTEMBER 9, 1999

Randy Rich, M.D., is the oncology fellow at Yale Medical School who primarily cares for me. Randy says, "This isn't a hospital, it's the set of a Disney movie!"

He's a hoot, and we banter mercilessly. For example, he says something funny and I quip, "An oncologist with a sense of humor, what an oxymoron!"

He shoots back, "A psychologist who isn't crazy, what an oxymoron!" When my humor can be this "sick," you know I'm feeling better!!! Love to you.

Was at Yale—could see Randy Rich coming my way out of the corner of my eye, and told my friend to ignore him, don't look! I sensed trouble.

"Hi!!" he stops in front of me, and says, "I need to take
you into an exam room."

"Why?" I ask, "Can't we just do it here?"

Now every patient in earshot is chiming in, and saying,
"Yeah, do it here!"

He says, "I don't think you want to do this here." So
we're in the exam room and he's talking a mile a minute,
just a tad nervous, "Cell counts are on the border, . . .
blah, blah, blah, . . . check for bleeding, . . . blah,
blah, blah, . . . transfusion, . . . blah, blah, blah,
 . . . arrange shots, . . . blah, blah, blah, . . .
rectal exam, . . . blah, blah, blah. . . ."

"What!" I think.

A short while later, after abruptly performing a rectal
exam, he says, "OK, I'm done."

"That was good," I say, "but will you call me?"

For the first time since I've seen him, he has no quick
comeback!

"Advantage!" I think.

In these last three lines we see Bette's humor. She flusters the
oncology fellow, throwing him off balance. He's speechless. By her
wit Bette has gained the upper hand. She comes away laughing, with
her dignity preserved. The alarming and humiliating situation has
been transformed into something to laugh about—an example of the
healing property of humor, which I mentioned at the beginning of
the chapter. Humor defuses tense situations and allows people to be
more human. With their playful sarcasm and friendly banter, Dr. Bette
Furn and Dr. Randy Rich have developed a wonderful relationship.

FEBRUARY 16, 2000

I went to Yale today. They had an advanced practice nurse
and a couple of patients talking about lymphedema. Now
this is something I very much want to know more about, so
I was looking forward to this. The nurse started out the

talk, and, frankly, from the get-go, I thought she wasn't
the sharpest pencil in the box. She was a couple of
flapjacks short of a stack, a couple of tracks short of a
CD; the elevator didn't go to the top floor. She gave just
straightforward information, like definition, description,
that sort of thing. Then she turned the discussion over
to the patients, who did a show-and-tell with the stuff
they use to counteract the swelling.

Lymphedema, in case you don't know, is a swelling of the
affected limb, from a buildup of lymphatic fluid that
can't move because the lymph nodes, their exit portal,
are gone [because the breast surgery removed lymph nodes
from the armpit]. So I'm thinking, before we get to show-
and-tell, and before the Benadryl kicks in and I get
loopy, I want to know a few things. Like, I want to know
what causes someone to get this, what are the odds. Give
me some numbers. What can be done prophylactically to
prevent this? Why not use some of those gizmos the
patients have before you get this, to prevent it, because
once you get it, you have it for life.

I came on strong, especially as the meds took over. I
don't think she liked me. "So deal with it!" I thought.

But she said stupid things, like, "You really don't need
to use the pressure bandages preventively. It's not
necessary." Then went on to say that a patient was flying
to China, and because this woman was going to be on a
plane for so long, they recommended she use a pressure
bandage even though she didn't have lymphedema, as a
preventive!

"Hey, Nancy nurse, didn't I just ask that?" I thought.
"And by the way, what was that about flying?" There was
absolutely nothing on her list of eighteen-things-to-do-
to-reduce-your-risk about the increased risk of flying!

There was something about not lifting more than fifteen
pounds with the affected limb. So I asked her about
playing tennis. I figured that banging a tennis ball
might qualify as strain.

"Oh, no," she said, "normal activity is fine."

But there were four people in the room with lymphedema,
and two of them had gotten it from exercise!—one from
running, and one playing racquetball.

"Hey, Nancy nurse," I thought, "you can understand that
this is not reassuring information? Can you see that?
That, basically, you can get lymphedema from pretty much
anything, or not, at pretty much any time, but maybe not.
Well, thank you, that was soooo helpful. Snore. . . ."

MARCH 16, 2000

Hello, everybody!!! Rise and shine, rise and shine! I've
been up for well over two hours, which puts me three mugs
of caffeine ahead of you, so get your cups and get ready
to chat. It'll be a little one-sided at first, but. . . .

Went to Yale yesterday. Seven visits down, five to go. I
had a whole list of issues I wanted to discuss: symptoms—
nosebleeds, unexplained bruising, the continued
neuropathy, too many bathroom trips (indelicate, but
true), memory problems, extreme fatigue, no appetite. I
had questions—why twelve weeks of this, why not eight or
ten or fifteen—and I want a compelling answer—something
better than "because"—because, if I don't get an answer,
I'm outta here. I want to know everything they know about
lymphedema, specifically, how not to get it—when should I
consider initiating a referral to a plastic surgeon, and
how does Dr. Restefo sound, he was suggested to me. I was
wondering if I should have the reduction on the left side
done first, or have it done the same time I have the
reconstruction done on the right. What do you think? Hm?

I got to pose all these questions to a new oncology
fellow, Dr. A _ _ _ _ . I'll always think of him as Dr.
Argue, which is what he did pretty much every time he
opened his mouth. He asked stupid, misinformed questions.
Here's a little tip for Dr. Argue: read the chart BEFORE
you see the new patient. And, you want to hear something
really scary? He'll be done, completely finished, with his
training in June!

Good Lord, help us all! He noticed my business card on
the pad where I had made my notes to myself, and said:
"You're the second psychologist I've seen today."

"Gee, no kidding," I thought to myself. "I wonder if
there's some reason they sent you to TWO psychologists!"
It just makes one wonder, don't you think? I want my old
oncology fellow back (Dr. Randy Rich). Think about it—
would you rather see Dr. Argue or Dr. Rich—it's a no-
brainer. Did I mention my memory problem? And does
anybody here know someone named Wayne, or maybe it was

Bonehead? I can't remember. Just a little inside humor—
which one of us won't be laughing at.

Anyway, then I saw Dr. Burtness, in all her usual,
efficient, pleasant glory. Basically she said, "Don't
worry about the bleeding at this point; stay on the same
Coumadin dose." The fellow wanted to cut it by two
thirds. "Don't worry about lymphedema, you had a very
good surgeon, you're very low risk." I need to know more,
though. She said more that I don't remember clearly.
"Your memory problem is a combination of chemo-brain
and menopause; it will pass. Talk to the plastic surgeon
about a week after finishing chemo; he won't talk to you
any earlier than that, and Dr. Restefo is who I'd want
working on me. I want you to try a low dose antidepressant for your peripheral neuropathy, and the other
symptoms." She went on with the medical rationale for
why.

I think part of what she was doing was using medical
reasons to get me to take an antidepressant. Because
along the way, I said, "and, it could help with
depression." She gave me that knowing nod. She's good
. . . real good. And, it's twelve weeks because research
data has shown that one month is insufficient, and six
months is intolerable (for most? for me? I don't
remember), so we settle on twelve weeks. Admittedly a bit
arbitrary, but an educated approach.

That's about all I can remember. And who are all you
people?

June 13, 2002

CT scans yesterday—all negative, so no internal spread to
the organs.

This spread over the skin is referred to as localized
breast cancer. (And I mean spread.) Low dose radiation is
raised as the best means of controlling that. So, it
looks like gamma knife, round two, here I come.

Optimists are pleased. The rest of us are merely
adjusting course.

The last line implies that Bette is not an optimist. After all, even if
the breast cancer has not spread to internal organs, any recurrence
is ominous.

DEATH ON MARCH 28, 2003

Bette Furn died at age fifty-two, leaving behind her daughter, Krista, age eleven; her son, Parker, age twenty-two; and her sixty-year-old husband, Peter Moody. A funeral service was held at St. Paul's Episcopal Church in Woodbury. At Bette's request the service was at night. After the service, many of Bette's friends and family stood and said a few words. It was very moving.

Rabbi Lawrence Silverman's Perspective

I asked Rabbi Lawrence Silverman about humor and sick people like Bette. He's been my friend since our undergraduate days together at Brown University, before either of us got our theological training, before either of us was ordained. For thirty years Lawrence has led Congregation Beth Jacob in Plymouth, Massachusetts. Much of his work is involved with chronic illness, primarily because of counseling members of his synagogue, for as you will see in the next chapter, about half the people in any congregation suffer from chronic illnesses. Lawrence also served on the ethics committee of several hospitals.

Lawrence said, "Over my years counseling people who are chronically ill, I've noticed that people who regain their sense of humor retain their connection to other people. They may not live longer. But they are less isolated and live more fully for as long as they do live. When sick people laugh, I've found that there is a reflective wisdom to it. Their laughter is not denial. It is how this person is connected to life and to other people. They are aware of the frailty of life."

His comment reminds me of Bette Furn, who remained connected to her friends through hilarious emails. As Lawrence, his wife Meredith Hoffman, and I discuss these things, we are having breakfast at Persy's Restaurant. I had drawn a cartoon of Meredith in college, and she thought it was so funny that she kept it forty years and brought it to show me at breakfast. Lawrence and Meredith are vegetarians. All of us had cornbread, home fries, and coffee.

"There is a midrash about the infertility of Abraham and Sarah," Lawrence says. "Sarah had been bitter and jealous of Hagar. When an angel comes to Abraham and announces that the couple is going to have a child, Sarah laughs. This is the key to understanding the name 'Isaac,' which in Hebrew is *Yitschâq*, which means 'one will laugh.' According to this midrash, it is the laughter that heals Sarah and lifts her out of infertility so that she becomes productive. I gave this as a Rosh Hashanah sermon, which is the time of year when this Torah passage about Sarah laughing is read.

"You are familiar, of course," Lawrence says, "with Norman Cousins's book on laughter.[1] As a matter of fact, I believe that the *Reader's Digest* column, 'Laughter, the Best Medicine,' is inspired by Norman Cousins's work on laughter as a way to deal with cancer."

If a person with cancer has friends, there is something wrong, namely the cancer. One way of dealing with the problem is to deny or hide it. In the old days, before Betty Ford and Happy Rockefeller went public about having breast cancer, women would never tell anyone that they had cancer, not even their sisters or closest friends. It was considered shameful. Women used to live a decade or two with breast cancer that no one else knew about. Things have changed dramatically during my lifetime, so that it is no longer shameful to have cancer, and people talk about it openly. Other chronic illnesses have not yet become as respectable as cancer.

But there is still a problem when a person with cancer has friends. How can everyone relate to each other without being overwhelmed with negative emotions, such as sadness, horror, fear, or pessimism? Is it safe to discuss the cancer, or should that subject be carefully sidestepped? It is awkward. Is it polite or impolite to mention it?

Humor provides a solution to these dilemmas, as we learn from Bette Furn and Rabbi Silverman. Laughter allows the cancer to be acknowledged without making it a problem that estranges the sick person from his or her network of friends. Humor is a social lubricant that makes relationships comfortable.

The Humor of Beverly VanGerud

We turn now to Beverly VanGerud, who lives in Florida and has a different style of humor. I said before that the humor of sick people may be hard to understand, because it tends to be dark and sarcastic, which insiders think is uproarious, but outsiders don't get it.

Beverly works for a large bank. Her lupus causes her joints to be inflamed and painful. One day, during a flare-up, she is too uncomfortable to get out of her chair to get a cup of coffee.

"Does anyone around here know that I have lupus?" Be
in a mocking tone of voice. "Is anyone going to make any co.

This comment sends her co-workers into hysterics. It is priceless.
"Here we go," one of them says as she gets up to make coffee. "We're
going to get the lupus routine again." More laughter.

"Yeah," chimes in another co-worker, "I think I need to get lupus!"

By using her sense of humor—and being willing to be kidded by
her co-workers—Beverly maintains a healthy connection to her fellow
employees at the bank. She may not live longer, but she lives more
fully because the humor allows her to have a vibrant relationship
with her co-workers.

"A joke means everything is okay," she tells me. "I want people to
be in their comfort zone. So I cover my problems with humor. Jokes
are camouflage."

Inside Beverly's merriment, however, is found the nub of the problem, how to convince herself things are okay when they aren't. How
do you make light of that which is heavy, or change lead into gold?

Bev has three medical problems:

- She has lupus, which causes arthritis that is so bad that she
  sometimes can't get to the bathroom because of pain in her
  joints, especially her hips. She has an unusual form of lupus
  that attacks her lungs as well. She gets pneumonia and can't
  shake it for months. That could be what will kill her someday.
- She has two tumors or hygromas growing on her brain. A
  hygroma is a localized buildup of cerebrospinal fluid (CSF).
  Normally a hygroma is found only in the brain of an infant
  or someone very old. It is called hydrocephalus and is treated
  surgically with a shunt. The tumors press on and displace Bev's
  brain. No one knows if they are malignant. To find out, neurosurgeons would have to do an operation, but the risk of stroke
  after surgery is so high that the surgeons and Beverly have
  opted to wait and watch the hygromas with an MRI every six
  months. Meanwhile the hygromas cause her to have crushing
  headaches and memory deficits. Only a few of her co-workers
  know about the hygromas.

- Bev takes dangerous medicines (Cytoxan and Plaquenil) that have potential side effects like blindness. Her co-workers don't know about these serious possibilities.

Suppose you are Beverly's co-worker. You know about the lupus and that periodically she is absent from work for eight weeks with pneumonia, because lupus weakens her lungs. You are confronted with a choice. Are you going to cry for Beverly or laugh with her? Beverly's condition is overwhelmingly sad, but she acts wacky and offers you the option of laughing. Fun is much more compatible with the task at hand, which is collections for the bank. If you were to allow yourself to appreciate the full force of the misery of Bev's lupus, you would be unable to get your work done. So when Bev offers you the choice of merriment, you jump at the opportunity. Thus, in context, these conversations are so funny that you love going to work with this heroic clown.

Beverly has figured out how to enable her co-workers to have a relationship with her and still get their work done. She is a magician who is able to turn heartbreak into lightheartedness, an alchemist who converts lead into gold.

Kurt Luchs, a writer of humor, attends my church. (His latest book has just been published: *Leave the Gun, Take the Cannoli: A Wiseguy's Guide to the Workplace*.) You met his wife, Suzanne, in chapter 1. Kurt says that the crucial factor in humor is "the frame." By this he means the context, the framework of assumptions and the narrative up until this point. Bev and her co-workers share the same frame, so it is easy for her to make jokes that they find hilarious.

Bev hates sympathy. Hidden inside sympathy is condescension. There is the covert thought, *I'm glad I am not you!* As far as Bev is concerned, it would be better to eat a slug and die than be subjected to the erosive acid of sympathy.

One day Bev's nonverbal cues made it evident that she was in agonizing pain. A co-worker said, "This must be a bad day."

Beverly wisecracked, "It depends on what day I feel I need attention." The co-worker laughed. That allowed Bev to laugh. Everybody relaxed.

Our heroine has learned to avoid sympathy by inviting other people into a fantasy world in which a make-believe tyrannical queen pretends to have lupus pain for the sole purpose of manipulating her co-workers so that they will pay attention to her. This trick allows the others to relax. Only when her co-workers are at ease can Beverly convince herself that excruciating hip pain is nothing. It is as insignificant as a mosquito bite.

Bev's ability to relax and put others at ease started when she was a teenager with a fabulous voice. She took singing lessons, had fantasies about going to Julliard School of Music, and sang in the church choir. But she had stage fright. It was no easy trick to stand up to sing a solo in front of an audience without seizing up with fear. Other people advised Bev to imagine the audience naked. Naked didn't work. But ridiculous hats did. Bev would imagine her listeners were wearing absurd hats and amusing plumage, thereby allowing herself to relax and sing.

Interaction was the key. "It is amazing how circular life is," Bev said. If Bev appeared to be relaxed, then the audience could relax. They preferred to enjoy the music rather than fear that the soloist would freeze. She could see it in their faces. Once the body language and facial expressions of the audience conveyed relief, Bev would be able to relax and sing. In a circular way, humor functioned to convince first Beverly, then the audience, and then Beverly again that things were okay.

Beverly has always been a people-pleaser, externally oriented since childhood. If everyone around her was happy, then she felt things were okay. The primary goal of her interactions was to put others at ease and make them feel good. That was the circuitous method by which she managed to feel good about herself. Four decades later she realized that the approach she had used when singing would work at her bank, when she was contending with tyrannical diseases.

Because of lupus, Bev's immune system is incompetent at fighting infections. Once Bev's breasts were infected and swollen. The infection was not responding to either antibiotics or surgery. Bev made a joke of it. "Dolly Parton gets a lot of attention because of the size of her breasts," said Bev. "So I'll be like Dolly."

When Bev began taking Cytoxan, a chemotherapy drug used in severe cases of lupus, there was a risk that her hair would fall out. Her sister Carole, who is a nurse, told her she should buy a wig in advance. Then she'd be prepared. Bev bought the wig but loathed it. She dealt with her revulsion by cracking a joke. She threatened Carole that if Carole's boyfriend found the wig sufficiently attractive, he might stay with Bev and not return to Carole. Everyone laughed, which made the wig less loathsome.

Bev's humor extends to her interactions with physicians. When a neurologist was advising Bev about the hygromas on her brain, he told Bev that she should go to get a neurosurgical consultation at Shands, which is a neurosurgical group associated with the University of Florida.

"Would you send your mother there?" Bev asked.

"Yes," the neurologist said.

"Let me ask you one more question," Bev quipped. "Do you like your mother?"

This question struck the neurologist as hilarious. As a result, he relaxed and disclosed more medical information than he would have otherwise.

Bev is a collections expert. "I'm a bill collector," she says. She has taught collections inside banks for twenty-five years. She knew the laws and regulations, but she was beginning to have trouble at work. She couldn't think. Important things were missing from her memory; everyday things that she'd known for years were gone. This was the effect of the hygromas compressing her brain and causing memory deficits. There was a risk that she might lose her job. Bev began carrying a notebook to keep track of information, such as the name of the person she had spoken with ten minutes earlier. At her bank you cannot make a mistake. The culture won't tolerate it.

"When people wonder why I can't remember obvious things," Bev says, "I say that I have water on the brain. They burst out laughing. I don't tell them that it is literally true, that I do have water on my brain. A few people at work know about my hygromas, but they think they don't bother me. My headaches are so bad that sometimes I want the doctors to amputate my head, but I don't say that to my co-workers.

"My faith in God gets me through," says Bev. "Many a night I lie awake asking God why he allows me to be sick and never feel good." When Bev gets down like this, she remembers her father's heroic struggle with cancer and how he never complained or blamed God.

"I brought this on myself," her dad would say, referring to his cigarette smoking. Her father's example allows Bev to relax and not challenge God. The issue with disease is not whether we know God's plan but whether we trust God.

Why Sick People Use Humor

When sick people can laugh, it means that the human spirit triumphs over the mean-spirited destructive powers of disease. Humor reflects the joy of resurrection, whereas disease is more akin to crucifixion.

Humor dethrones disease—which has a way of controlling a person's life—and places the person in control. It converts that which is dull and gruesome into something dazzling, imaginative, and outrageous. It ridicules the emperor named "disease" for having no clothes and therefore restores dignity to those crushed by that emperor.

You might not think that chronic illness, folderol, and tomfoolery could commingle, but they can! If a disease tyrannizes you, mocking the disease restores human dignity. One way of dealing with insoluble problems like breast cancer, lupus, and hygromas is to turn the problems inside out and upside down. By force of humor you can so distract your mind from the disease as to upset the apple cart and bemuse the spirit. In that way you can rescue yourself from paralysis of the will, so that everyone can relax and use their best judgment.

As illogical as humor may be, it is nevertheless more logical than disease. In grammar a double negative equals a positive. "We don't disagree" means "We agree." Similarly it seems that the irrationality of disease is negated by the irrationality of humor, resulting in a restoration of sanity. Whereas disease is bad news, humor reminds us that our long-term biography in God's scheme is good news. Comedy triumphs over tragedy.

This Form of Humor in Literature

The humor that sick people enjoy is often sardonic and derisive. The very nature of this humor is that it draws a boundary line between the insiders who think it's funny, and the outsiders who think it is weird and not the least bit funny. This style of humor can be found among other groups of people who suffer afflictions they cannot control, such as slaves, oppressed minorities, or soldiers in combat.

The Uncle Remus fables, enjoyed by African American slaves in the United States in previous centuries, used irony and satire to make a mockery of whoever or whatever was oppressing the slaves. In these stories Brer Rabbit gets the best of Brer Bear, who is far more powerful but stupid. This is the humor of the underdog.

The humor of sick people is like the humor of the Old Testament, which was written by slaves and an oppressed minority.[2] Consider the book of Esther. There is a mocking tone toward the villain Haman, who plans genocide of the Jews. Exaggeration is used to heighten the irony—the gallows from which Haman is hanged is seventy feet tall (Esther 7:9–10). Outsiders don't think that hanging is a laughing matter, but insiders throw a party every year, called Purim (see 9:18–32), to celebrate the fact "that the evil scheme Haman had devised against the Jews [came] back onto his own head" (Esther 9:25). Unless you are Jewish and celebrate Purim, chances are the book of Esther does not seem amusing to you, which defines you as an outsider. And that is my point.

Sick people in our time likewise ridicule the tyrannical disease and other forces of oppression, such as managed-care companies, unsympathetic healthy people, drug side effects, and a variety of other sources of harassment. It is like the Roadrunner mocking the Coyote in a cartoon, or Brer Rabbit being so smart and sassy that he once again makes a fool of Brer Bear.

Another kind of humor that may seem out of place is that of soldiers in combat. Paul Fussel, author of *Wartime: Understanding and Behavior in the Second World War* and *The Great War and Modern Memory*, says that in a war troops develop a black humor as the only way to deal with the insanity and horror of the battlefield. They sarcastically portray the battle scene as an absurd comedy staged by the president or generals. Gallows humor keeps them from coming unhinged.

One example is Joseph Heller's book *Catch-22*, which is about the efforts of an airman named Yossarian to save his own skin in Italy during the closing months of World War II. A catch-22 is the rule that every rule has an exception. In other words, there are no rules and nothing makes any sense, including war. The law governing war is without rhyme or reason. It can be depicted as an absurd comedy.

My point is that black humor is well known in literature and is characteristic of slaves, soldiers, and anyone who is downtrodden by preposterous situations that they cannot control. Such derisive humor is based on the frame, as Kurt Luchs says, but only the insiders who share that same frame of reference think it is funny. A core characteristic of most of the humor of sick people is that outsiders don't understand it.

The Humor of Jack Less

Everyone differs in what they think is funny. Bette Furn and Beverly VanGerud use sarcasm, but Jack Less uses more traditional jokes. His humor is gentle, kind, and not sarcastic.

Jack Less is an eighty-seven-year-old retired businessman who lives with his wife Rose (age eighty-three) in an apartment on Fifth Avenue in Manhattan, overlooking Central Park. He is perpetually smiling and cracking jokes, which keeps the mood light. People love having him around, because both he and Rose are delightful.

"It is my wife who is so gregarious," Jack says. "We've been married sixty-five years. She is bubbling and supportive. We have three grandchildren and four great-grandchildren."

For decades Jack and Rose had a sign on the kitchen wall about the three Cs of marriage: commitment, communication, and compromise. Rose underlined the word *communication*, because Jack didn't talk much at the beginning of the marriage. Over six decades she taught him to talk, or at least that's her version.

They both came from poor families. Jack's dad sold shoelaces and razor blades in Manhattan. Neither Jack nor Rose could afford to go to college. They married when she was eighteen, and over the course of their marriage they've had a lot of excitement.

Jack founded a company that manufactured hairbrushes. He made more than a billion of them during his career—one million new hairbrushes a week from 1945 until 1991. Chances are you've used a brush made by All American Brush, Jack's company.

I visit Jack and Rose's apartment on a cold, rainy day in May. Jack is wearing old jeans and a plaid shirt and looks completely healthy. Rose is wearing a simple dress. They are thin, fit, smiling, and gracious. Both of them look to be twenty-five years younger than they are.

This illustrates something that I will talk about in the next chapter, namely that old people aren't "old" anymore. They are "young." They think of themselves as young, have young friends, and act young.

Both of them encouraged me to write this book, *Being Sick Well*, because they know so many friends who could be helped by it. By their mid-eighties, many of their friends have a chronic illness and a few have died.

Jack and Rose are relaxed and delighted that I have taken the time to visit with them. They show me around. Their apartment is full of beautiful pieces of art, including several things that Jack collected over the years, such as statues of elephants. One wooden elephant is four-and-a-half feet tall, a massive presence. The apartment is spacious and has plenty of room for such an imposing sculpture.

Jack's humor and positive attitude make it easy to forget that he has serious medical problems. "As long as you can laugh at it, it's alright," Jack says.

"Years ago Rose and I came up with the formula for a long life," Jack says. He pauses, waiting for me to ask what it is.

"What?" I ask.

"We get one day older," he continues, "every week." Again he pauses, waiting for me to laugh. He joins me in laughter and says, "It's nice work if you can get it." He keeps laughing.

Meanwhile I'm thinking, *So this is why old people aren't "old" anymore!*

The problem is that Jack is sick. A quarter of a century ago Jack had a malignant melanoma removed surgically from his shoulder. Then he had bowel problems requiring surgical removal of six feet of his intestine and five hospitalizations. Seven years ago he had coronary artery bypass surgery and a mitral valve replacement. The ejection fraction of his left ventricle dropped to 12 percent. A normal heart should push more than half of the blood out into the aorta with every heartbeat. At 12 percent Jack's heart isn't pumping much blood. He has atrial fibrillation, severe heart failure, an internal pacemaker, and automatic defibrillator. Jack also says he is "loaded with arthritis," in his shoulders, ankles, and fingers. He has gout and osteo- and rheumatoid arthritis. He takes six pills in the morning and fourteen in the evening and goes to a cardiac rehab gym three days a week for a vigorous workout, walking as much as he can on the other days.

"It is six and a quarter miles around Central Park," Jack says. "I used to run it. Now I walk, but not nearly that far. Yesterday I was walking but I was so stiff from arthritis that I had to stop after a mile. I felt stifled. The key is perseverance. If it hurts too much to walk today, I go out and try again tomorrow. It's faith that keeps me going. You have to believe you can do it, and you have to believe that God has his eyes on you so that you are going to get better. If it hurts, then I do it again. With all the medical problems I've had, I've never believed I wouldn't make it."

"Faith is very important to Jack," Rose says. "But he doesn't talk about it much."

"I think it is easier to have faith if you have lived a good life," Jack says. In the Manhattan business world, Jack Less had a reputation for honoring his commitments, never ripping anyone off, never lying, and always paying his bills. "I have always tried to be ethical. If I'd deceived people or cheated them, then I don't know if I would be able to be so comfortable with my faith."

Jack and Rose belong to five synagogues. Usually they go to the Park Avenue Synagogue, a conservative congregation in Manhattan. They also belong to a conservative temple in Brooklyn, another in the Garment District in Manhattan, and a temple in Connecticut near their daughter, plus they contribute to an orthodox synagogue in Morristown, New Jersey, that rescues kids from drug addiction.

"They don't just belong to these synagogues," Jack's son-in-law tells me. "They also work the crowd. They give of their time and money and know the rabbis well."

For decades Jack and Rose raised money for an organization called Cancer Care and for Israel. Rose had lost her mother to cancer and had a bout with breast cancer herself.

But I'm rambling. You, no doubt, would like to know more about Jack's contribution to this chapter on humor.

"We're having the time of our lives," Jack says. "We are able to take life as slow or fast as we want. We go to every new Broadway play and musical, every new ballet and opera. We love to go out to meet friends in a restaurant. The only problem is that I had to stop driving four years ago because I get dizzy. Rose and I get along well in every respect except that I'll never get used to her way of driving the car. We've lived a good life because of faith and humor."

"When did your humor start?" I ask.

"Well, I was born at an early age." Jack pauses, waiting for me to laugh. "My humor has never left me. If I'm on my back on a stretcher in the hospital, I tell a joke to the people around me. I have hundreds of medical jokes. If I'm hurting, telling a joke interrupts the pain and allows me to get some relief. Jokes have helped my attitude. The other day I was at a doctor's office and I told a joke to the girls behind the desk, and they laughed. Their laughter raised me a few inches off the ground. It keeps me from dwelling on things."

His comment reminded me of Beverly VanGerud, who uses humor to connect with other people and to distract herself from her medical woes.

"What is your best medical joke?" I ask.

"Hmm," Jack ponders, "I have so many of them. I don't know if I can tell you the best, but I can tell you the most recent. A man goes to the doctor and says, 'Doctor, Doctor, you have to help me. When I touch my neck, it hurts. When I touch my chest, it hurts. When I touch my stomach, it hurts. Everywhere I touch, it hurts. When I touch my thigh, it hurts. You have to help me, Doctor! What are you going to do?'

"The doctor says, 'Well, I'm going to have to get X-rays of your entire body and maybe some scans.' Later the doctor comes back and says, 'I've figured out what is wrong with you.'

"'What?' asks the man.

"'You have a broken finger,' says the doctor."

Jack pauses for me to laugh, which I do. Then he swings into the next joke.

"Years later, when he's old, the same man goes back to the doctor's office and has a complete physical exam. Then the doctor says, 'Now I'm going to need a sample of your stool, a sample of your urine, and a sample of your blood.'

"But the man doesn't hear very well. 'What did you say?' he asks. The man turns to his wife and asks, 'What did he say?'

"His wife says in a loud voice, 'He says that he's going to need a sample of your underpants!'"

"That's an interesting joke," I say.

"Since you're a psychiatrist," Jack says, "I've got one about a psychiatrist. A man takes Viagra. But he's having the runs. So he goes to his psychiatrist and says, 'Doctor, I'm taking Viagra but I have the runs.' So the psychiatrist asks, 'What do you take the Viagra with?' 'Prune juice,' the man says. 'I swallow my Viagra with prune juice.' So the psychiatrist says, 'I know what is wrong. You don't know if you are coming or going!'"

Jack goes on to tell me how he and Rose deal with the problem of communication between his doctors. Because there are so many doctors involved, Rose came up with a brilliant idea. Twice a year the couple invites all the doctors and their wives to dinner at a restaurant. The doctors and their wives love it. This keeps the doctors on a first-name basis with one another, thus facilitating communication between them concerning Jack's medical condition. Jack and Rose love socializing, especially at a restaurant that is quiet enough for them to carry on a conversation. Rose used to be a food critic for a New York magazine, so she knows the owners of many Manhattan restaurants.

"So, we're sitting at dinner," Jack smiles, "and I tell these doctors that I'm going to tell them a joke that will test their medical knowledge. We get a magazine from the Mayo Clinic, the Cleveland Clinic, the Lahey Clinic, and Harvard Medical School, so I'm up on the latest medical developments. So I tell them I'm going to tell a joke that will test their medical knowledge."

"Oh no," Rose says, squirming, "not that one!" Rose is politely making fun of her husband's propensity to tell jokes. The affection between them is palpable. They work well as hosts, putting a visitor like me at ease. Rose serves a delicious berry tea, along with crackers and a jar of almond butter from Israel.

Jack is not deterred. He tells his joke: "A boy is born with a silver screw head in his belly button. The pediatrician shrugs it off and says he doesn't know what it is. Specialists examine the child and say they've never seen anything like it. Over the years other kids, especially in the locker room in gym, torment the boy because no one else has a silver screw head in his belly button. When he gets to be a man, he's still troubled by his condition, so he goes to leading doctors, and they examine him, shrug their shoulders, and say, 'I don't know what it is. My advice to you is to ignore it!' But the man can't ignore it. He's obsessed. So he journeys to India to a leading guru and discusses the problem. And the guru tells him that he knows how to cure the condition. He tells the man to go on one specific day of the year to Egypt, at such-and-such time of day to kneel in front of the biggest pyramid and pray.

"The man has to wait eleven months for the specific day that the guru had said. So he goes to Egypt and kneels before the biggest pyramid just at sunset. He's kneeling there and it's getting dark and he wonders, *Now what's going to happen?* No sooner does he think that than a bright light appears at the top of the pyramid, no bigger than a pinhead, and a beam of light radiates down and shines on the man's belly button. Then he sees that there is a glove inside the light, and the glove comes forward from the apex of the pyramid, and comes down inside the shaft of light. The glove gets closer, the man sees that the glove is holding a silver screwdriver. And the glove and screwdriver come closer and closer, until the screwdriver fits inside the slot of the screw in his belly button. The man sees that there is a perfect fit between the blade of the screwdriver and the slot in the head of the screw. Then the glove begins to turn the screwdriver. As it does, the screw unscrews and comes further and further out of the man's belly until it is entirely out. Then the glove and the screwdriver, with the screw attached, withdraw up the shaft of light and back into the bright spot of light at the top of the pyramid. Then the light goes out. So the man is still kneeling there in the dark at the foot of the pyramid in the sand. And he's thinking, *Now what?* He kneels there, squatted on his haunches for a long time, waiting. Nothing more happens. Finally, he decides it's time to go. So he stands up. And his rear end falls off."

I laugh.

"So I've told the doctors that this joke will test their medical knowledge," Jack says, laughing.

Unlike the ridicule and sarcasm of Bette Furn's and Beverly VanGerud's humor, Jack's jokes lack the biting edge that I had thought was characteristic of the humor of sick people. He comes across as a peaceful and caring guy who loves to crack a joke. He seems less tortured than Bette or Beverly. I have to keep reminding myself that Jack's life dangles by a thread. In no way does he look sick. He and Rose are so charming and cordial, and they look so young and vigorous that it is hard to remember the magnitude of Jack's medical disasters. When I talk with Rose alone, though,

I am aware that the precariousness of Jack's life is always on her mind.

"When we get on the elevator in our apartment building," Jack says, "I always have a joke to amuse the elevator man. I pretend to be involved in forty different businesses. If it is raining outside, I say the weather is great because I'm in the umbrella business. If it's snowing, I say it's great because I'm in the ski business. If it is sunny, I tell him that I'm in the sunglasses business. He always laughs when we ride the elevator. Of course, it's all fiction."

As we relax together, Rose tells Jack to show me one of their most cherished possessions. Their nephews and grandchildren had a clock made by Tiffany's. Inside the mahogany box is inscribed a plaque to "Meeps," which is an affectionate name for Grandpa. The inscription reads, "Your vision, strength and love spawned a legacy of promise, creativity and integrity for generations to come. For the seeds you have sown, the world is a far better place. No one could have done more. With love and respect for your inspiration, Scott, Andrew, Adam, Jason and Melissa." I am touched that Jack and Rose trusted me with such an intimate appraisal of what the grandkids think of Meeps.

Jack and Rose have a vast social network—strategy one for dealing with chronic illness. They have friends scattered all over New York City.

"We are the rarity," Jack says. "I was born in Manhattan and I've lived here my whole life. Everyone else is from somewhere else. We had a house on Long Island and a house in Connecticut in addition to this place. Our house in Connecticut was on Candlewood Lake and had 6,500 square feet, including a full-scale bowling alley and a swimming pool in the basement. It was right on the shore of the lake, great for parties. When we were doing so much for charity, we'd bring busloads of people up to Candlewood Lake for a weekend."

Because of his business, Jack has close friends in Korea and Taiwan, in Taipei. He manufactured hairbrushes in the United States but imported raw materials from Asia. He is godfather to many children in Asia, where he has gone sixty times on business trips, always with Rose. The couple has so many friends in Israel, France, England, Italy, and scattered across the United States that they have a problem scheduling visits. For example, they have been invited to three weddings on the same day, and they can't fit in all three.

"Our life is good," Rose tells me, "providing we don't have to make any more trips to the Orient, or schlepping all over the world. I'm getting worried. Jack is slowing down in recent years. I suggested that perhaps it was time for him to show me the books so I would know about things, but he said there was no need for that yet. I don't know what makes someone like Jack so upbeat while other people are beaten down by their illnesses. I do think that a good marriage is a big part of it, and we have had a very supportive marriage, even though there have been some heartbreaks. Every day with Jack is special.

"I think you should tell your readers," Rose continues, "that when you get to be our age, even with all the illnesses, sex is still important." She and Jack smile. "Sexual activity still goes on and is still an important part of marriage. Affection and enjoyment continue. I think your readers should know that."

Strategy Seven: Take One Day at a Time

Deborah Chase says she tries to live one day at a time. This doesn't mean that every day is a good one. It means that she focuses on the here-and-now rather than the future. One day I wanted to talk with Debby, but she wasn't at her home when I dropped by. I found her in the intensive care unit of my hospital with unstable angina. She was waiting for yet another cardiac catheterization.

"You can see why I live one day at a time," she told me. "I don't know when I'll have the cardiac cath, and when I do, it depends on what they find whether they transfer me to another hospital or keep me in this one. Nothing is ever clear about the future for me."

Unlike Jack and Rose Less, Debby lives on the brink of poverty.

"I live one day at a time," she continues, "because I believe everything happens for a reason. You may not like the reason. But God always has a reason that is good for you. People get upset with me because I refuse to worry about the future. Like one day I wanted to move from one state to another, and people told me I wouldn't make it because I had no transportation, job, housing, or money. I just went to church and prayed. Within twenty-four hours someone offered me a truck. I had a job lined up and an apartment. Someone gave me enough money to make the trip. So I just trust God. He doesn't fail me. That's why I can forget about tomorrow and worry only about today!"

Like Bette Furn, Beverly VanGerud, and Jack Less, Deborah is able to find life amusing. Her conversation is punctuated with belly laughs that are contagious.

She is fifty-one years old. She uses her last name, Chase, as a nickname.

Looking at Chase, people wonder if she is a fraud, because she doesn't appear to deserve her disabled license plate. She looks healthy, but when she walks a short distance, she gets chest pains and shortness of breath. She has so many health problems that I hardly know where to begin.

Chase has anti-thrombin-III disease, as well as some form of lupus. Therefore she has repeatedly suffered from:

- blood clots causing strokes, heart attacks, and cardiac arrest
- emboli, which are the hand grenades tossed off from clots, such as TIAs (transient ischemic attacks) or pulmonary emboli
- side effects of medicines to prevent clotting, such as massive bleeding in her intestine or hemorrhagic stroke

Chase takes a dangerous combination of blood thinners. At the time I interviewed Chase, she was taking fourteen powerful medications every day: amiodarone, amlodipine, atorvastatin, clopidogrel, digoxin, enoxaparin, eptifibatide, furosemide, lisinopril, metopolol, nitroglycerine, pantoprazole, warfarin, and zafirlukast.

"At age forty-six I had a bad year," Chase says, chuckling. "I was in the hospital every month, usually around the first of the month," she laughs. "It got to be a joke. Dr. Dobkin, my cardiologist, said that if I didn't get better, he would take me out back and shoot me. My problems were giving him an ulcer. That was hilarious. That year after having a heart attack, stent, and open-heart surgery, my gall bladder went bad. Surgery was needed. Dr. Dobkin said, 'Debby, your gall bladder?' That was hysterical. It meant, 'What else could possibly go wrong? Your gall bladder isn't even related to anti-thrombin-III disease!'"

Dr. Dennis Dobkin, a cardiologist, treats many patients with crippling disease and often wonders whether he would be courageous or crushed if he had similar problems. He put me in touch with Chase.

God only knows how Chase got anti-thrombin-III disease. Although it appears to be a genetic problem, no one in her family has it. The whole thing arises from one specific biochemical error, namely a malfunctioning of the molecule anti-thrombin-III. She has five healthy brothers and sisters. "I'm the lucky one," she says. And there, in that quip, you see again a glimmer of her humor. She giggles with a sincere cheerfulness.

Deborah is so good-natured that she has repeatedly had a problem communicating with doctors. They tend to underestimate the gravity of her symptoms. At one point, when she was having trouble breathing, her doctor assumed it was just anxiety. He prescribed a tranquilizer and told her she was being a baby and complaining too much. In reality Chase had a collapsed lung. That was in the days before she met Dr. Dobkin.

Once she went to the emergency room feeling as if someone had hit her on the head with a hammer. The overworked emergency room physician wanted to send her home because she was "just another case of a headache," but her friend refused to take her home. The doctor was harried because there was a heat wave and the emergency room was packed. Only after Chase had been ignored for eight hours and had lost her vision did the doctor realize that this headache was different. Chase had had a hemorrhagic stroke.

Debby tells me with humor, "That's the advantage of taking three powerful blood thinners. After strokes, because your blood is too thick, you get to experience a stroke because your blood is too thin.

"I suppose I don't complain enough," Deborah says, laughing. "I mean, really, what is the point of complaining? For the most part it serves no purpose. I can't stand people who whine! If you complain or you are terrified, what difference does it make? Usually there is nothing anyone can do about it anyway. If you are going to have another heart attack or stroke, it doesn't matter whether you complain or don't. So why complain? It's pointless! That's what I say. Besides, if you complain, pretty soon no one listens.

"No matter how bad your disease," Chase continues, "there is always someone worse off. That other person might be heroic, selfless, and completely good-natured, like this woman with lupus who shared a hospital room with me. She was the most delightful person I ever met. She had these terrible ulcers on her legs. She saved my life one day. I got out of bed to tell the nurses that my stomach discomfort was getting pretty bad. The nurses had been ignoring me and telling me that I should stop griping about a minor stomachache. I vomited a huge amount of blood and fell under the bed, unconscious! My roommate called for help. That saved my life."

"I can see that you are prepared to die tomorrow," I say. "How do you manage to remain so calm?"

"Me?" Chase replies. "Die tomorrow? No way! I'm not ready for that! There are too many things I want to do. I've been president of the PTA and chairman of the newcomer's club, sung in the choir, taught the junior high church school, been president of the twins' club. I've been in charge of Meals on Wheels and on the school advisory council. I'm not ready to die tomorrow! Who would take care of my eighty-eight-year-old father if I died tomorrow? As a matter of fact, I don't even have time to waste being sick.

"I have a strong belief in God," Chase continues. "That is what gets me through all this." She doesn't talk much about her faith. It is simply part of her assumptions about life. As I listen to her, her meaning becomes clear. She isn't worried about tomorrow because she is in God's hands. It is up to him, not to her, whether she has another stroke, heart attack, or some other disaster. God is kind. All she has to do is trust. For that reason, she remains relaxed. God has never failed her. So why worry? Life is an amusing adventure.

When I ask Chase to elaborate on how faith has taken her through these troubled waters, she deflects the question and talks about peripheral issues, like her denomination, the choir, and church school. She doesn't directly and explicitly tell me how God has pulled her through the tough times. This reminds me why doctors so often underestimate the importance of faith. People like Chase or Jack Less don't talk about their daily interactions with God. It is simply part of life. They are practicing strategy nine.

Squirrel Metaphor

Once when I was looking out the kitchen window, I saw a neighborhood cat chase a squirrel from our yard across the grass and up an oak tree. The cat stood at the bottom of the tree, swishing her tail, agitated. Suddenly the squirrel jumped down on the grass, near the cat, and ran across the yard again, toward a second oak tree, with the cat in hot pursuit. The squirrel made it.

That squirrel was just messing with that cat's mind! It was exhilarated by tempting death and outrunning the cat by an inch. Why else did the squirrel jump onto the grass a second time?

Chase is like that squirrel, exhilarated at outwitting death, escaping annihilation by the breadth of a cat's whisker. She is different, though, because mostly she doesn't put herself in harm's way. I say "mostly" because, until four years ago, she smoked cigarettes. Aside from that she does not jump down on the grass near the cat.

Her attitude is more like this: If you find a cat chasing you, what are you going to do? Some people freeze from intimidation, and the cat swallows them. Others are motivated by hatred of the cat or they run out of mortal terror. Chase treats the race as a game. That may be why she has the nickname Chase. Her motto could be, "I outrun the stupid cat ten times out of ten!"

If you don't make a game out of staying one step ahead of death, then the chase gets very old very fast. By keeping one step ahead of death, Chase ridicules the grim reaper and shows that her spirit is frisky and not about to succumb.

Chase appears to be indestructible. Except for some memory deficits, she has recovered from three strokes. And her heart is still pumping against all odds, with an ejection fraction about as low as that of Jack Less. She looks pretty good, considering that she is a veteran of so many wars.

"When doctors say over me that I'm not going to make it," says Chase, "I ask myself, *Who are they talking about? Not me!* Doctors are all gloom and doom. No one thinks positive. I always pull out of these near-death experiences and do just fine! It would be better if the doctors were optimistic."

Chase never thinks about tomorrow. She lives in the present. Tomorrow is of no interest to her. Her refusal to worry about the future reminds me of the New England Centenarians Study that I heard about from Dr. Tom Perls in Boston. He is studying people who are one hundred and older. He says they have a relaxed attitude about the future, even in the face of a 50 percent per year mortality rate. Much of their calm acceptance is due to spirituality, he finds. They say they are in God's hands. Furthermore, they have weathered so many storms that they are accustomed to heavy weather. Their attention, much like Chase's, is on their children and grandchildren. They don't focus much on themselves. Most of the centenarians have children who are full of vitality at age eighty, and energetic grandchildren who are sixty.

A Series of Questions

The moral of Chase's story is that it is beneficial to be positive and live in the present moment. Jesus taught: "Do not worry about tomorrow, for tomorrow will worry about itself. Each day has enough trouble of its own" (Matt. 6:34).

I want to understand Debby Chase better, to see clearly how she manages to live one day at a time. So I ask her a series of questions. I ask her what it would be like if she worried about next year.

"Why would I do that?" she replies, puzzled. "I don't worry about the future for myself or my children." There is a long silence. I finally realize that she has said all she is going to say.

"Do you make any future vacation plans?" I ask.

"No," she says. "We can't afford vacations. Besides, I'm more of a spur-of-the-moment person. I go and visit family, but I don't plan it ahead of time."

"Is there any advantage to living one day at a time?" I ask.

"I never thought about it," she replies. "I just live that way. That's just the way life is. I don't worry about what's going to happen tomorrow. Tomorrow could change in the next twenty-four hours anyway."

"If you have a really bad day," I ask, "do you hope that tomorrow will be better?"

"No," Debby says. "I just *know* it will be better. I can depend on it. I don't need to hope that it will better."

"Do you have life insurance?" I ask. I am probing to try to figure out how thoroughly she is committed to not worrying about the future.

"No," she replies.

"Do you have a will?"

"No."

"Looking back over your life," I say, "would you do anything differently, change some of the decisions you made?"

"I never looked back," she replies. "I guess if I think about it, I would change some of the clothes I used to wear. Sometimes when I look at old photos, I wonder, *What were you thinking?*"

"What would you see as your greatest accomplishment in life?" I ask.

"My children," she replies.

"What do you regret the most?"

"I regret that I've not been as healthy as other people," Debby says. That seems like an understatement to me.

I am left with the impression that Debby Chase is a straightforward person who simply lives life as it presents itself, without comparing herself to anyone else and without worrying about tomorrow or yesterday. She looks and sees how things are. Then she accepts them, knowing that she is in God's hands. That is simply how life is for Debby. She lives out the Alcoholics Anonymous motto: "One day at a time." In the process of living the way she does, Debby finds life filled with joy, and she is an inspiration to people around her. Others, like her cardiologist, Dr. Dobkin, view her as courageous and fun to talk to.

"Do you know that you bring sunshine into the life of Dennis Dobkin?" I ask.

"I do?" she sounds astonished. "That's news to me. He is really a neat person."

Once, when Dennis and I were both signing medical records in our hospital, I asked him what it is like to take care of Deborah Chase.

"Deborah has a mysterious upbeat attitude," Dr. Dobkin replies. "I can't imagine where she gets the gumption to bounce back with a smile on her face. She has real spunk. I am awestruck with her laughter.

"Deborah's laughter is different," Dennis continues. "When I say to someone, 'How do you manage to carry on amidst all these troubles?' people often laugh or snicker. They are embarrassed by the question. They don't know what to say. It can be a threatening question if you are dreadfully sick. But when I ask Deborah that question, she laughs and says something intelligent in response. From that I know that her laughter is genuine. She is amazing! I can't tell you, Jeff, how Debby manages to remain so good-humored despite having so many problems. Somehow she has avoided being bitter or angry with everyone. Her laughter is genuine."

"With all these medical disasters that she goes through," I say, "with all the times doctors have said she would not survive, doesn't Debby sometimes get depressed?"

"I've seen Deborah depressed, perplexed, and bewildered," Dennis replies. "But she rallies. No matter how desperate the situation, she always bounces back and becomes jovial and lighthearted before very long."

Conclusion

Imagine a world governed by an absolute rule that everyone must be healthy. But, catch-22, there is an exception to that rule. You happen to be an exception. You have a disease, which, mysteriously, is neither lethal nor curable. So the rule is that everybody is supposed to be healthy, except for you. All diseases are supposed to be either lethal or curable, except for yours, which somehow defies the curative power of medical science. There is something absurd here, don't you think?

How are you going to live with such a preposterous situation? This chapter has proposed two solutions to the paradox. The first is to laugh at how ridiculous it is; the other is to forget about tomorrow and squeeze all the juice you can out of today.

4

BAD NEWS AND GOOD NEWS
ABOUT THE EPIDEMIC

As I said in the introduction, this book has two themes. The first is that some sick people live well, and we can learn by listening to them. The second theme is that there is an increasing amount of chronic illness, the largest epidemic ever.

In this chapter we will consider the second theme. Near the end of this chapter we will return to the first theme, when I discuss the eighth strategy—exercise.

Many readers can't stomach statistics. They simply want to read the case histories illustrating the twenty strategies. If you are such a reader, you can skip to the case history of Gordon Lewis, two-thirds of the way through this chapter. This is the only chapter in the book that is primarily statistical and academic. I will try, however, to make it interesting reading, even for those who would rather eat a slug and die than to wade through statistics. In this chapter you will read about wolves, caribou, and Charles Darwin's survival of the fittest theory. You will read about an adorable seventy-three-year-old grandmother with gold teeth and neon orange hair, about having your friend amputate your leg in her kitchen, why you should do aerobic exercises and lift weights at age seventy-six and swim daily at age one hundred and one. It is even possible that you will enjoy this chapter!

There is bad news and good news about the epidemic of chronic illness. The bad news is that there is indeed an epidemic involving half the population, and it is getting worse over the decades. The good news is that there are decreasing disability rates among the elderly.

The Bad News

In the introduction I listed the three reasons this epidemic is getting worse. I also said it is a mystery that this epidemic is so little recognized, even though it is the biggest thing happening in health today.

Edgar Sydenstricker and the Effect of an Aging Population

Starting in the twentieth century, chronic diseases have become increasingly common. The first person to notice this was Edgar Sydenstricker in his 1933 essay "The Vitality of the American People." He noted that the infectious diseases were coming under control, and the population was therefore living longer. Up until then infectious diseases had been the primary causes of death. However, the American people were not enjoying the vitality that would be expected from longer life because the risk of heart disease, cancer, diabetes, stroke, and a myriad of other diseases increased with age.[1]

The epidemic is now more advanced than it was in Sydenstricker's day because the average person today is one or two decades older. Figure 2 shows that the risk of chronic illness increases as you get older. In this graph you can see that 24 percent of the youngest age group (ages 0–19) have at least one chronic illness, such as asthma or a skeletal deformity. As you move to the right, to older ages, the height of the bar increases. For people age sixty-five and older, 84 percent of them have one chronic illness; 62 percent have two or more.[2]

Figure 2 also contains information about comorbidity—having more than one disease. The white part of each bar shows the percentage of people who have just one chronic illness, whereas the black part shows the percentage with two or more chronic illnesses. The graph shows that, if young people have a chronic illness, they tend to have just one diagnosis. As people grow older, they tend to acquire additional illnesses. Someone sixty-five or older is more likely to have several chronic conditions, so that the right-hand bar has lots of black and not much gray.

Comorbidity is an important economic issue. People who have five or more chronic illnesses consume two-thirds of the Medicare budget.[3]

Figure 2

Prevalence of Chronic Illness by Age

*(percent of each age group
that has a chronic disease)*

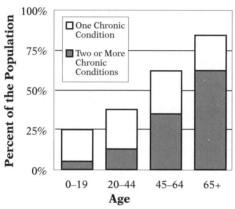

Data from Partnership for Solutions, *Chronic Conditions* (Baltimore: Johns Hopkins University, 2002), 11

Simultaneously the entire population is aging. I don't just mean that you and I are getting one year older every year, but the average age of the population is increasing. The primary reason for this is that the birth rate is so low. A secondary reason is that people are living longer, so the age group over the age of eighty-five is the fastest growing segment of society. When the entire population is aging, it means that everyone is drifting to the right on figure 2, with the result that there is a slow but steady increase in the amount of chronic illness and in the amount of comorbidity in every technologically advanced nation on earth.

This might give you the impression that most people with chronic illnesses are elderly. That is not the case. Most of the people with chronic illnesses are between the ages of twenty and sixty-four, and lots of them are younger than twenty. Less than a quarter of those with a chronic illness are age sixty-five or older. It is a misconception to think that chronic illness affects only elderly people.[4]

Ernest Gruenberg and the "Caribou Effect"

After Sydenstricker's essay, the next major paper on the subject was Ernest Gruenberg's talk when he won the Rema LaPouse award of the American Public Health Association in the 1970s. Gruenberg's famous speech, "The Failures of Success," proposed that people were surviving longer with chronic illnesses, and therefore those illnesses were increasingly common. Gruenberg spoke of how death was cowardly and tended to kill people who were frail and sickly at a higher rate than those who were healthy. Therefore, when we reduce the death rate, we differentially increase the survival of people who are frail and sickly more than we increase the survival of people who are healthy.[5]

Think of the relationship between wolves and herds of caribou. Caribou are sometimes called reindeer and are related to deer. They live in herds of hundreds of thousands on the tundra of northern Canada, Alaska, Scandinavia, and Siberia, feeding on grass, lichens, small shrubs, berries, mushrooms, twigs, and bark. A century ago, when there were many wolves, they killed off the frail and sickly caribou, which kept the herds strong, youthful, and healthy. A healthy caribou can outrun a wolf, and both wolves and caribou know this. Usually a wolf won't waste energy pursuing a healthy caribou, except as a test to see if the caribou has an invisible chronic illness and can't run very fast. Wolves hunt the most vulnerable caribou—the infants, old, chronically ill, or injured. It is generally agreed that without wolves the caribou herds would be sicker than they are when wolves are plentiful.

I will use the term *caribou effect* to refer to the idea that a caribou herd gets sicker when there are fewer wolves around. This is because the caribou with genetic defects and chronic diseases have a better chance of survival when there are fewer wolves to attack and kill them. The caribou effect is my way of explaining Gruenberg's "Failures of Success" paper. The analogy is that humans are the caribou, and killer diseases such as bacterial pneumonia are the wolves that used to keep the human population strong and healthy.

When my daughter, Felicity, was a child, she was delighted when I read her Farley Mowat's hilarious book *Never Cry Wolf* as a bedtime story. This is about Mowat's adventures as a naturalist observing wolves in the Canadian arctic, near the Hudson Bay. Mowat befriends an elderly Inuit named Ootek, who is wise in understanding wolves and caribou. They sleep in the same tent. Ootek tells the ancient Eskimo fable about how and why wolves were created. It seems that in the beginning there was a Man and a Woman and nothing else. The Woman dug a hole in the ice and pulled out all the different animals, including the caribou. Humans began to hunt caribou, but they preferred to kill the fat, healthy, and strong ones. Soon almost all the fat, strong caribou were gone, leaving only sick and weak caribou, which were no good for food, nor were their skins any good for clothing. The humans began to starve. So the Woman called Amorak, the spirit of the wolf, to prune the caribou herds by killing off the sick and weak caribou, so the herds would become strong again. As the herds got stronger and healthier, the humans had plenty to eat. The Eskimo realized that the wolf and the caribou were one, because the wolf feeds on the caribou, but the wolf also keeps the caribou herds healthy.[6]

Now what happens when breakthroughs in medical science allow us to kill off wolves, such as bacterial pneumonia? According to Darwin's theory of "survival of the fittest" (which I will discuss in a few paragraphs), we would expect the human population to grow older and sicker, just as the caribou do in the absence of wolves.

I remember my first experience of the caribou effect. When I was a third-year medical student at the University Hospital in Cleveland, a woman in her seventies was admitted with pneumonia. She had a high fever, labored breathing, and was barely conscious. A chest X-ray showed a white cloud in her lungs, and we stained her sputum and found bacteria. We made a diagnosis of bacterial pneumonia and rapidly got rid of that wolf by means of intravenous antibiotics. A few days later, when her fever was gone, the woman's breathing was comfortable. But she had almost no language and no memory whatsoever. We wondered what had happened. Had the fever somehow destroyed her mind? It was a mystery. We phoned the nursing home where she lived and found that she had been profoundly demented for twenty years. She had no family. Since her pneumonia was cured, we shipped her back to the nursing home. A century earlier this frail caribou would have died. Here we can see what Ootek told Farley Mowat, namely that when we doctors use antibiotics to chase away Amorak, the spirit of the wolf, more caribou with Alzheimer's and other incurable diseases survive, and, as a result, the human population gets sicker.

Gruenberg said that reductions in the death rate by killers such as pneumonia directly translate into a sicker human population stricken with incurable diseases like schizophrenia, Down's syndrome, spina bifida, and diabetes. He proposed a paradox: Better medical care can make a population less healthy. Gruenberg's paper on this subject is one of the classics of medical literature, often cited by experts discussing the epidemic of chronic disease.

A good example of the caribou effect is AIDS (see figures 3 and 4). Now that we have effective anti-AIDS drugs, we have turned AIDS from a lethal into a chronic condition. In figure 3 you can see that there are fewer new cases of AIDS and fewer deaths per year than at the height of the epidemic in 1992–1995. Between prevention and antiviral medicines, we are getting rid of the wolves. You might say we are winning the war against AIDS in the United States.

Figure 3

New Cases and Deaths from AIDS

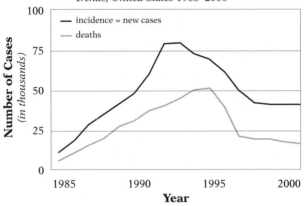

Trends, United States 1985–2000

Data from Centers for Disease Control website at www.cdc.gov/hiv/graphics/ images/L207/L207-17.htm

Figure 4

**Number of People Living with AIDS
as a Chronic Disease**

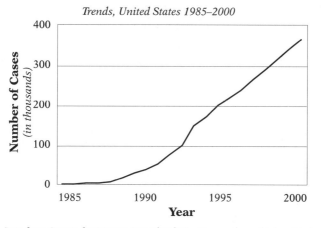

Trends, United States 1985–2000

Data from Centers for Disease Control website at www.cdc.gov/hiv/graphics/
images/L207/L207-17.htm

What is the impact of all this success in terms of the number of people living with AIDS in the United States? That is shown in figure 4. There is a progressive increase in the number of people living with AIDS, the number rising linearly and steadily, from less than 5,000 people in 1985 to more than 350,000 people in 2001, a rise of more than 7,000 percent. That's because we can prevent death from AIDS but have no cure for it. No one infected with the HIV virus ever gets rid of it entirely, so in that respect you could say that we are losing the war against AIDS in the United States.

Figure 4 demonstrates what Gruenberg said, that medical break-throughs sometimes result in more people with chronic, incurable diseases; because terminal illnesses are turned into interminable illnesses. When we lower the death rate, the people we rescue from death are more likely to be people with chronic illnesses, so that lowering the death rate usually increases the rate of chronic illness.[7]

There are other examples of the caribou effect. Cystic fibrosis used to be rapidly lethal. Today with good treatment a person can survive with that disease for decades. Now that more people are surviving heart attacks, some of them are going on to develop heart failure as a chronic condition, and that disease is increasingly evident in our hospitals.[8] Now that more people survive brain injury, an increasing number are living with cerebral palsy,[9] stroke, or TBI (traumatic brain injury). Effective treatment transforms cancer from a lethal to a chronic disease. Insulin allows diabetics to survive and lead productive lives, but as they live longer, they increasingly suffer the long-term destructive effects of diabetes, as in the case of my first wife.

Charles Darwin's "Survival of the Fittest"

What we are dealing with is one of the most basic laws of nature. Charles Darwin spoke of "survival of the fittest." Under adverse circumstances, when there isn't enough food or water, when there are epidemic plagues and natural predators, the fittest members of a species are more likely to survive than are the ones with chronic illnesses. That is classic Darwin.

What is less often recognized is the mirror image of Darwin's survival of the fittest law. What if agriculture improves so there is enough food, if engineers build reservoirs and pipe water dozens of miles to the city so there is enough water, if there are good sewers and garbage collection and therefore fewer epidemics, if people in the north have warm houses so less of them freeze to death, and if medical science reduces the number of killer diseases? The answer is that the population of humans begins to age, and more people with chronic illnesses survive. One day someone says, "Why do we have this increasing epidemic of chronic conditions?" The answer is, "Because, as strange as it may seem, conditions have improved."

When facing predators, bitter cold, and risk of starvation in the wild, caribou have a life expectancy of four years. If you remove the wolves and take care of the caribou in a humane setting such as a zoo, the population begins to age and lives as long as eighteen years. They also have more chronic diseases.

The same is true of domestic cats. They live a decade longer than their wild cousins but tend to have chronic diseases. We have two cats that are brothers, age fourteen. Phthalo has low thyroid and Alizarin has chronic heart disease. So you might say, "Look, I understand that you are saying that more humane treatment leads to increases in the rate of chronic disease in many species, but what kinds of names are those for cats?" The answer is that I named the cats after my favorite oil paints. We also have a younger white cat named Titanium.

The caribou effect, then, is the converse of Darwin's law of survival of the fittest and is responsible for the aging of the population. Darwin's law prevails when conditions are harsh (not enough food or water, so lots of death), whereas the caribou effect prevails when conditions are humane (abundant food and water, and less death). They are two sides of the same coin.

Systematic Studies of the Epidemic

There have been only two systematic studies examining the prevalence of all chronic diseases for all ages. Both were based on data from the Medical Expenditure Panel Survey (MEPS).[10] This survey provides diagnoses based on physicians' examination, using the *International Classification of Diseases, 9th Revision* (ICD-9). Using data from 1987, Catherine Hoffman and her research team classified each ICD-9 diagnosis as being either a chronic disease or not.

Hoffman showed that ninety million Americans had at least one chronic disease, which was 45 percent of the noninstitutionalized population of the United States.[11] That study provoked a lot of skepticism. Critics doubted that the numbers could be so high. They pointed out that Hoffman was only a nurse and said physicians were needed to make reliable diagnoses.

Therefore a research team led by Gerard Anderson at Johns Hopkins undertook a second study to replicate Hoffman's findings, using the 1996 MEPS data. Careful attention was paid to diagnosis. Two teams of physicians from Johns Hopkins Medical School, one being internists and the other pediatricians, went through the ICD-9 and classified each diagnosis as being either a chronic disease or not a chronic disease. The expectation was that with more attention to the diagnoses of chronic illnesses by academic physicians, the number of Americans with chronic diseases would be lower than what Catherine Hoffman had found. Quite to the contrary, Anderson's research team found even more people with chronic illnesses—one hundred and twenty million Americans.[12]

The studies by the Hoffman and the Anderson teams are important because they count people who are in treatment for a chronic condition as well as those who are not in treatment. Consider research on blood pressure, for example. High blood pressure is the most common chronic condition and is increasing in prevalence. The National Health and Nutrition Examination Survey (NHANES) through 1992 showed that if you went into a community with a blood pressure cuff, you would have found that blood pressure was falling in the United States in recent decades. It would have been a mistake to conclude, however, that there was progressively less hypertension, because such a research approach ignored the majority of people with a diagnosis of hypertension whose blood pressure was normal only because they took medicine for high blood pressure. They still had chronic hypertension. The prevalence of undiagnosed hypertension in America is 16 percent. A 2003 study by Hajjar and Kotchen based on NHANES data confirms that hypertension is increasing in the United States.[13]

What we need and don't have is a study of this epidemic over time, confirming table 1 (p. 20) that there is a slow but steady increase in the prevalence of chronic illness. Few researchers are interested in the kind of megaissues on which this book focuses. Research money from the National Institutes of Health is available to study specific diseases but not to study the trends in aggregate data for all chronic diseases combined. Therefore there are insufficient data to definitively answer the simplest questions facing our people today:

1. Is our population getting progressively healthier or sicker over the decades?
2. Are we winning or losing the war against chronic disease?

When insurance companies compare their data over a period of years, they find that there are progressively more diagnoses per insured person, more chronic diseases among young people, an increasing number of different doctors per person, an increasing number of prescriptions per person, and therefore rising costs because of this epidemic.

The Dawn of Chronic Disease Epidemiology

This chronic disease epidemic is well known in science and has caused a change in the way scientists conduct business. Take epidemiology, for example. In 1849, when Dr. John Snow studied the distribution of the cholera epidemic in the city of London and found that the illness was correlated with polluted water, the scientific study of epidemics began. The science of epidemiology is defined as the study of the distribution of a disease in a population and of the risk factors affecting that distribution. From the time of Snow until World War II, epidemiology focused on infectious epidemics, such as cholera, tuberculosis, small pox, malaria, yellow fever, syphilis, whooping cough, salmonella, influenza, and polio.

After World War II the population was living longer, so that chronic diseases replaced infectious diseases as the primary health problems. A new branch of epidemiology—chronic disease epidemiology—began. The most famous such study was the Framingham Heart Study, which discovered the causes of heart disease: high blood pressure, obesity, high cholesterol, lack of exercise, animal fats, cigarettes, and type A personality.

As our population continues to age, the chronic diseases become more widespread, so that almost half the population lives with one chronic disease or another.

I was trained in chronic disease epidemiology at the Yale Medical School's Department of Epidemiology and Public Health, and I served for seven years as a physician-epidemiologist in the Center for Epidemiological Studies at the National Institute of Mental Health, in Bethesda, Maryland.

Invisibility of the Epidemic

Although the epidemic of chronic illnesses is the most massive thing occurring in healthcare today, it tends to be a silent issue, one that is not talked about as much as it needs to be. In part this is because of the way medical practice is organized. Our entire medical financial system is set up to pay for short-term (acute) episodes of illness and is not designed to pay for chronic conditions or chronic care. Our patterns of practicing medicine prevent us from thinking about problems that don't fit into our organizational and bureaucratic structure.[14]

John Inglehart (a leader in American health policy and editor of *Health Affairs*) writes, "Chronic health conditions . . . afflict an estimated 100 million Americans. But, ironically, chronic illness is largely absent from the national health policy agenda."[15]

The deficiencies of the medical system vis-à-vis chronic illness are documented in the Institute of Medicine's book *Crossing the Quality Chasm: A New Health System for the Twenty-First Century*. This highly influential book points out that the current medical system cannot do the job required of it and that trying harder will not work. Only changing the way in which medical care is delivered will improve the quality of care.[16] Thomas Bodenheimer and colleagues have also published articles on this subject.[17] These people tend to criticize the medical system for ignoring chronic illness, but the reimbursement system (the insurance companies and government) do not structure their payments so as to encourage any change in the system. We are locked into a system, now costing Americans 1.7 trillion dollars a year, that is not good at responding to the needs of the majority of patients—those with chronic illnesses.

Every doctor and nurse I know is aware that the epidemic of chronic illnesses is *the* major unsolved problem in conventional medicine, but few people are talking about the magnitude of the problem. This is the elephant standing in the middle of the living room that people politely don't mention. One reason they don't mention it is because we can't really acknowledge the size of this elephant without overhauling the way we pay for medical care and the way our hospitals and medical schools are organized. The entire medical system will need to change. For example, disease management companies, such as American Healthways, Encompass Health Management Services, Integrated Wellness Solutions, or Landacorp, often do a better job dealing with chronic illnesses than do conventional doctors, but if you talk to physicians about disease management, they don't comprehend what you are talking about. "We are already doing that," they say. They don't see that disease management is a different kind of care.

What is disease management? It starts by identifying those patients who have expensive or chronic illnesses in a population. By "a population" I mean, for example, those people who are insured by a particular health insurance company. Computers track the behavior and healthcare costs of such patients, and case managers then try to develop strategies to contain or reduce those costs. For example, if a patient is repeatedly hospitalized, the case manager would try to make sure that the person goes to office-based follow-up appointments with his or her doctor to become more stabilized outside the hospital. The case manager might make sure the patient has a cheap or free supply of medicines at home to manage the disease. The case manager could phone the patient daily to see how things were going and find out if the patient is compliant with treatment. Computers track whether such interventions result in lower costs. Innovation is possible for patients who are high utilizers, such as getting a visiting nurse to go to the patient's home seven days a week or paying for intravenous treatments at home. If a patient with a potentially expensive diagnosis, such as bipolar disorder, does not refill his medicines on schedule, the disease management company learns this from the pharmacy computer and sends a letter to me (the patient's doctor) alerting me to a possible lapse in compliance, so I can phone the patient and deal with the situation before the disease flares up and leads to another twenty-thousand-dollar hospitalization.

While the motivation of a disease management company is cost containment, the result is improved treatment of the disease. Large employers or health insurance companies pay for disease management because it reduces the total healthcare budget.

Disease management companies criticize traditional medical doctors, saying that they are not *patient focused* but are *appointment focused* in their treatment. The emphasis in a doctor's office is to make sure the appointment book is scheduled and to see everyone in the waiting room. Of course, when people don't show up for appointments, they are usually people who need special attention because their noncompliance leads to disease flare-ups and repeated hospitalizations, which are expensive.

Traditional doctors criticize disease management companies for focusing on only one disease at a time, such as the management of diabetes, while ignoring the complexities of real life in which patients often have a half-dozen diseases and need a personal relationship with their physician to establish trust and become reliable quarterbacks on the healthcare team.

In reality there is no competition between disease management companies and physicians. We work collaboratively as partners dealing with some patients who consume the lion's share of the health-care dollar. Some of these patients are stubborn and difficult people who don't like having a disease, don't like treatment, and don't want to cooperate with anyone.

Case History: Shiqirije Silvia Krosi

The following case history illustrates another reason that the epidemic of chronic illness is invisible. The story is about Shiqirije Silvia Krosi, a seventy-three-year-old Muslim woman who lives in Waterbury, Connecticut, where I work.

Shiqirije (pronounced shi-KEER-ee-ya) was born into an Albanian family living in Yugoslavia. Her father forbade her to go to school, because she was a girl, and when she insisted, he beat her with a belt. Her father prevailed, so Shiqirije never learned to read or write. She had four brothers and two sisters. Only her brothers attended school.

At age sixteen Shiqirije entered an arranged marriage with a seventeen-year-old Albanian boy, Adem Krosi. It was a good marriage that lasted thirty-seven years. The couple settled in Albania, just across the border from Yugoslavia. Then the Communists took over Albania at the end of World War II. Adem hated the Communists. Within three years the couple risked being shot in an escape across the border in the middle of the night with their baby, even though Shiqirije had not wanted to make the attempt because of the risk of being killed. After the escape they lived in a refugee camp in Yugoslavia for five years, hoping the Communists would be thrown out of Albania so they could return. Alas, Communism persisted for decades.

Adem and Shiqirije migrated to France where Adem worked in a factory and became a central figure in the Albanian community in that part of the country. He helped Albanian refugees find jobs. During their twenty-three years living in France, Shiqirije raised their seven children and a garden. She made sure that both the girls and boys had a good education. Today her children live in France, Italy, Sweden, and the United States. She has eleven grandchildren and one great-grandchild.

When Shiqirije was forty-seven, she and Adem migrated to Waterbury, where there was an Albanian community and three mosques.

The monetary exchange rate was good, so they were able to buy a house in the United States. Six years later Adem died.

Shiqirije continues to live a quiet life in Waterbury. You would never notice her except that she dyed her white hair bright orange, brilliant like the setting sun, with henna, a dye that is used by elderly Muslim women. The color enhances the gold fillings of her teeth so that the entire picture is luminous. "My family keeps the traditions of our culture," says Shiqirije's daughter. "So my mother is like an Albanian museum."

Shiqirije loves to talk about politics. Her view is that Osama bin Laden and al Qaeda are not Muslims. She can't stand them. They should not be associated with Islam, which is a gentle religion that respects individuals. They are simply criminals and should be eliminated, she says. Shiqirije loves democracy. She likes having a separation of church and state. Religion is a personal matter concerning one's family life. She would never want to live in a Muslim nation where they would restrict whether a woman shows her ankles. Her desire is to be a good American and a good Muslim, which are compatible goals to her mind. If she were forced to choose loyalties in a conflict, her loyalty would be to the United States.

As Shiqirije has aged, her health has begun to fail. She developed high blood pressure, asthma, and arthritis. Her knees ache almost all the time, but Motrin helps.

These are not catastrophic illnesses, but they are long-term illnesses—the topic of this book. Chronic illness means long-term conditions, and these illnesses are what most doctors spend most of their time treating. These are common diseases. High blood pressure is the most common chronic condition, with asthma and arthritis following close behind.

Often we don't recognize how extensive this epidemic of chronic illness is, because we have catastrophic illnesses in mind when we think of an epidemic. If we stop looking for the wrong thing and begin looking for conditions such as hypertension, asthma, arthritis, and diabetes, suddenly we realize that chronic illness is everywhere around us, affecting half the population. Just think how many people you know who take pills, use inhalers, or rely on herbs for one health defect or another.

Shiqirije's children convinced her that exercise would help her arthritis. They bought her a treadmill. Ten minutes a day she walks on the treadmill, despite the pain, and is slowly increasing the amount of time she walks. It hasn't helped yet. Mostly, for the past six years, she has been resigned to living with pain, but she bears her affliction with dignity. From Shiqirije's viewpoint, pain is a gift from God. It is his way of reminding her that her body is not eternal. Death is inevitable.

Shiqirije's medical conditions are not obvious and are a relatively minor but annoying part of her life. And this is typical of many Americans. Her diseases mean that she has lived a long and rich life and has acquired the diseases that come with aging.

More Reasons for the Invisibility of the Epidemic

There are many reasons for the invisibility of the epidemic of chronic illness. We have discussed two reasons so far, namely that the entire medical system has trouble acknowledging that which doesn't fit into its organizational structure, and we think of catastrophic illness when we think of chronic disease.

Most people with chronic illnesses continue to work and do not appear to be sick. Consider Dr. Arvind Patel in chapter 1, a skilled cardiologist who never mentions his cancer; or Dr. Bette Furn, Beverly VanGerud, or Jack Less in chapter 3, who were powerhouses of productivity at their respective jobs. Chances are you do business with people like them and never know they are sick.

Your co-workers may take medicines for high blood pressure, asthma, or diabetes, or they may persevere silently while suffering from sleepless nights caused by bad backs. People are proud and don't want to admit they have problems. They would feel diminished if they talked about being in the doctor's office last month, so they don't mention it. Life is more enjoyable if you don't dwell on your illness (strategy three). Therefore we may be incorrect when we assume our neighbors are healthy.[18]

Another reason the epidemic is invisible is because when we do talk about chronic diseases, we are trapped by our diagnostic system—the ICD-9. I am one of the coauthors of this diagnostic system,[19] so I am well aware of its many advantages and strengths. But ICD also has disadvantages. It balkanizes our thinking about chronic diseases. It divides and conquers us. Families taking care of a child with cerebral

palsy fail to recognize how much they have in common with families taking care of someone with Alzheimer's, namely the burden of
caregiving. We fail to recognize how much a child with many birth
defects, such as Zachary Sowle in chapter 1, has in common with a
retired person with five diseases, namely the burden of a healthcare
system that is biased against chronic care and health insurance that
refuses to pay one doctor to spend time being team leader. As a result medical care is uncoordinated and doctor A doesn't know what
doctor B is prescribing.

Our diagnostic system is superb for classifying individual trees. It
leaves us blind to the ecology of the entire forest. This book is about
the growth of the forest. I am interested in the trends of aggregate data
over a period of decades. One of my teachers said to me, "Jeff, your
way of thinking is unusual because you try to think things together
into a unity, while everyone else is using their mind to tease things
apart into separate entities." Since the epidemic concerns the growth
of the entire forest, and our diagnostic system restricts us to focusing
only at specific species of trees, we tend to be blind to the epidemic.

LACK OF COMMON CAUSE

In my city there is a fundraising campaign organized by the
American Cancer Society called the Relay for Life Walkathon. People
pledge money to sponsor volunteers and the number of miles they
walk. I gave five dollars last week. There is no similar fundraising
campaign for chronic diseases in general. The American Lung Association responds with a billboard downtown that says, "Fighting
big tobacco, bad air, and the asthma epidemic." The American Stroke
Association has a notice in the bathroom of my workplace, increasing
my awareness of stroke. Then along come the people raising money
for juvenile diabetes, Lou Gehrig's disease, Parkinson's, and dozens
of other chronic diseases, one diagnosis at a time. The world is full
of competing diseases, all trying to get your attention, all asking for
a financial contribution. If your family member has one of the diseases that win in this competition (such as heart disease or cancer),
then you don't see any problem, because you are supporting one of
the popular diseases. But if your family member has a rare disease,
such as chronic osteomyelitis, you discover that few people have any
interest in raising money or public awareness to help you.

What is lacking is a sense of common cause among the different disease constituencies. If the families afflicted with diseases X, Y, and Z would cooperate instead of competing with one another, there would emerge an advocacy group representing a majority of the public, and suddenly the healthcare finance system would be forced to change so as to recognize and treat chronic illness. That would make life with chronic disease much more tolerable for everyone.

This shows how our diagnostic system has made us blind to the common issues. ICD-9 has turned various diseases into competitors and left us blind to the fact that "different diseases present common problems and allow common solutions," as Gerard Anderson of Partnership for Solutions says.

If you go into a bookstore, you find the same thing. The shelves devoted to "health" are divided into hundreds of books focused on one particular diagnosis per book, all in alphabetical order. There are no books focused on the big picture of all chronic illnesses combined.

Unlike many preachers, I try not to repeat myself. But just this one time I'm going to violate that rule and reiterate something: "Different diseases present common problems and allow common solutions." Here is an example. Carol Youle is a librarian here at Waterbury Hospital. She has a bad back. Health insurance is happy to pay tens of thousands of dollars for back surgery but refuses to pay a few hundred dollars for physical therapy to prevent deterioration of her back so she can avoid future surgery. This is another problem that people with chronic illnesses face, regardless of diagnosis.

Our diagnostic system tends to blind us to the common human elements that people with disease X have in common with those with disease Y. There are common human reactions and triumphs that span a multitude of diagnoses. Someone learning to live successfully with heart disease has much in common with someone who is learning to live successfully with cancer, diabetes, depression, arthritis, or breathing trouble. We need to learn from and support each other.

What Leaders in the Medical Field Won't Tell You

There is one final reason that the epidemic of chronic illnesses is invisible and not talked about, namely that leaders in medicine avoid mentioning it. Medical opinion leaders promote this media message: "People are getting healthier and healthier because of breakthroughs

in medicine."[20] The charter of the National Institutes of Health speci-
fies that their medical spokespeople are to lobby for government
funding and taxpayer support to pay for advances in medical research.
The media message, "People are getting healthier and healthier,"
arises out of this charter, which does not include a responsibility to
focus on the financial consequences of breakthroughs in medicine
or to talk about the epidemic of chronic illness.

This media message has been effective, in the sense that Congress
recently doubled the budget of the National Institutes of Health. Medical
research is a multibillion-dollar business vital to our medical schools. It
is big business on the stock markets of Wall Street, Tokyo, London, Paris,
Frankfurt, and Toronto. Because of this media message, the discoveries
of Catherine Hoffman and Gerard Anderson get pushed to the sidelines
and ignored, because the idea of an epidemic of chronic illness doesn't
square with the message that we are getting healthier and healthier.

It's true that today children with congenital heart disease are rescued from death by surgery, which, of course, I applaud. This is
consistent with the media message that medical research is leading
to greater health, which is the viewpoint that medical leaders want to
keep in the forefront of our consciousness. But then comes the other
half of the story. Many of these children continue to have complex
cardiac problems for the next thirty-plus years. As they grow up, these
little survivors may need as many as ten cardiac surgeries over the
course of five decades. This vital medical intervention requires twice
as many healthcare dollars as other cardiac patients.[21] The cost of
this care puts a further burden on an already weakened healthcare
system. The central theme here is that our healthcare system lags
behind the advances used in saving these children.

Medical opinion leaders don't address this side of the financial equation because it is not part of their mission. Their half of the equation is
to save lives. They are successful when they obtain more tax dollars to
save lives through research and development. The news media focus
on the message that people are getting healthier because of medical
research, and tend not to report the epidemic of chronic illness.

More and more people are wondering if we can afford all this
high technology medicine. If you have a chronic disease and must
choose between preserving your nest egg so your children can go to
college or paying for a medical "miracle" that will give you another

six months of life, is it reasonable to spend all the money on medical treatment? The epidemic of chronic illness calls for us to redefine healthcare and fix the system so there is more fairness and justice. It is not right that working people have to go into debt to pay for medical treatment and forgo paying for cars, houses, churches, charities, vacations, and their children's education. In chapter 9 you will meet Janine Jacobsen who may die when she turns sixty-five if Medicare won't pay for the intravenous feeding that sustains her life.

Impact of the Epidemic

Although the chronic illness epidemic is invisible, the impact of the epidemic is highly visible, namely increasing healthcare costs. As I said before, people with chronic illnesses account for 78 percent of the healthcare budget today,[22] and they are increasing as a proportion of the population as well as a proportion of the budget.[23] The total amount of medical costs, hospitalization costs, out-of-pocket medical expenditures, and prescription drug costs rises dramatically with the number of chronic illnesses a person has. Someone with one chronic illness consumes twice as many healthcare dollars as someone with no chronic illness. If the person has three chronic diseases, the ratio is seven times as many dollars, compared to someone with no chronic illness. If the person has five or more chronic illnesses, the ratio is fifteen.[24] Thus it takes only a tiny increase in the rate of comorbidity to produce a large increase in the total healthcare budget.

The cardinal symptom of chronic illness is pain in the pocketbook radiating to the wallet. "People with serious chronic conditions report numerous difficulties paying for care. Some declare bankruptcy, while others borrow from family or friends to pay for care."[25]

Figure 5 shows a projection of how chronic illness will drive up healthcare costs in future years. The basis for this projection comes from the 1996 MEPS data. Direct medical costs are expected to more than quadruple over thirty years, based solely on the effect of the epidemic of chronic illness powered by the aging of the population.[26] This is not counting the effects of other expensive issues such as the fact that new drugs and technology are more expensive than older drugs and older technology.

Figure 5

Direct Costs of Chronic Illness in Future Years

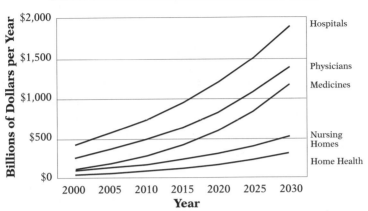

Data from Sin-Yi Wu and Anthony Green, *Projection of Chronic Illness Prevalence and Cost Inflation* (RAND Corporation, 2000), 17–23, tables 11–17

Let me devote this one paragraph to a discussion of managed care. This is an approach that has been used in the United States since the 1990s to try to put the brakes on rising healthcare costs. There are two interpretations of what managed care means, and they have diametrically opposite effects on the welfare of patients with chronic illnesses. *Capitation* payment is usually beneficial to the chronically ill. Since the chronically ill consume the lion's share of the budget, capitation leads to efforts to provide excellent care to them, so as to control the most important economic variable. But almost all other managed care strategies (other than capitation) lead to efforts to shortchange the chronically ill by disallowing services and cost shifting, because the chronically ill consume the lion's share of the budget. This ends my discussion of managed care.

Every nation faces the problem of skyrocketing healthcare costs. Today healthcare consumes 15 percent of the Gross Domestic Product (GDP) in the United States.[27] During my lifetime I expect to see healthcare costs soar to 25 percent of the GDP, so that one quarter of my income will go toward healthcare as I get older.

We are getting less and less for the money we spend—we have less time with our doctors and pay larger copayments for medications.

Forty-three million Americans have no health insurance at all, and that number is increasing as Medicaid and Medicare get into worse financial trouble. The future of healthcare finances looks bleak, and the injustices are getting worse.[28]

Two friends of mine, Sue Gearhart and Emily Littman, were joking with each other about how we are getting less and less medical care for our dollar. Sarcastically they said that by the time they get old, they expect that if you need a leg amputated, the insurance company will probably mail you a saw and an instruction book for how to have a friend do it in your kitchen. More sick humor that helps us cope with insoluble problems.

The Good News

Are you ready to hear some good news? The good news I'm about to tell you amounts to a different way of thinking about the epidemic. Despite the rising tide of chronic illness, there is a decline in the level of disability among the elderly. Thus, although more people than ever have chronic illnesses, those diseases may be less devastating than the same diseases would have been for our grandparents. That could be the key to understanding the epidemic in a more optimistic way. Later in this chapter I will tell you about experts who are even more optimistic than I am, primarily because of the decreasing rates of geriatric disability.

In 1977 Ernest Gruenberg predicted that people stricken with incurable diseases like Alzheimer's, schizophrenia, Down's syndrome, spina bifida, or diabetes would, as they got older, slowly overwhelm our civilization (the caribou effect). Twenty years later Kenneth Manton discovered that there was a decline in the level of disability among people aged sixty-five and older. This means that reality is not as simple as Gruenberg predicted.

Kenneth Manton's data are so famous and have had such a major influence that we need to talk about his findings (figure 6) in some detail. This graph shows trends of disability among persons sixty-five and older. All three lines of the graph are sloping downward as you go from left to right, and that is the main point.[29]

- The top line on figure 6 shows that, in 1982, 14 percent of the elderly population had trouble with one or more Activities of Daily Living (ADLs, described in the introduction); by 1999 that number had declined to 12 percent, if you use age-adjusted data.

- The middle line on figure 6 shows that, in 1982, 7 percent of the elderly were in nursing homes and other institutions. By 1999 that number declined to 4 percent, based on age-adjusted data.

- In 1982, 6 percent of the elderly who were free of ADL difficulties had trouble with Instrumental Activities of Daily Living (IADLs). These are activities related to independent living such as managing money, shopping, preparing meals, doing housework, or using a telephone. By 1999, that number declined to 3 percent, as shown in the bottom line on figure 6, which, again, is based on age-adjusted data.

Figure 6

Disability Decline among the Elderly

(ages 65 and older, United States, 1982–1999)

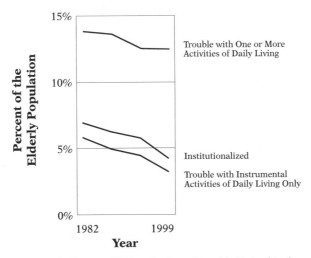

Data from Kenneth Manton and XiLiang Gu, *Proceedings of the National Academy of Sciences* 98, no. 11 (May 22, 2001): 6357, table 2

Other researchers, using different data sets, have replicated many of Manton's findings.[30]

You may be confused because figure 1 (in the introduction) showed a trend toward increasing rates of disability among children and working-age adults, but figure 6 shows a trend toward decreasing rates of disability among the elderly. The explanation is that disability rates are getting better for the elderly but worse for the young. There is need for more research to understand why these trends are going in opposite directions, but it appears that old people no longer think of themselves as old and therefore are more likely to act like young people. Jack Less (in the previous chapter) says that he and Rose have decided to grow just one day older every week. Both of them look twenty-five years younger than they actually are. They are like dynamos in terms of their level of activity.

Successful Aging

Researchers are discussing a new concept called *successful aging*.[31] It relates to an individual's ability to take an active role in maintaining his or her health. "Perceived self-efficacy, the belief that an individual can alter his or her own health future, is powerfully associated with health."[32] Jack Less is an example. He has learned that exercise is essential and goes frequently to a cardiac rehabilitation program at the YMCA or else he walks vigorously in Central Park.

Shiqirije Krosi is another example of an old person being younger than old people used to be. She is more independent and capable than she would have been if she had lived fifty years earlier in Yugoslavia. If she had lived then, she would not have lived alone at age seventy-three nor would she be the head of the house. Other people would have done the shopping, cooking, and housecleaning. Clearly Shiqirije likes being the boss, because her children offered to have her live with them, and she said, "No thanks!"

Here is how I think about the situation today. Two opposite things are happening simultaneously: First, there is a worsening epidemic of chronic illness, and, second, old people are no longer "old." Children and middle-aged people are more disabled because of the trend toward more and more chronic illness. The same would be true of the elderly, except that they are not aging as fast as they used to. The more youthful old people are, the more likely they are to overcome the tendency toward disability. Jack and Rose Less look and act as vigorous as sixty-year-olds, even though Jack is eighty-seven and Rose is eighty-three. Recognizing that old people are younger than they used to be, our government has increased the retirement age.

A few years back my mother, who is ninety, and I agreed that she should move from New Jersey, a hundred miles away, to live closer to me. She now resides in an assisted-living facility nearby. In that facility she is considered one of the young people. Mayo Okada, originally from Japan, is one of my mother's neighbors. Ms. Okada just celebrated her 101st birthday.

As I mentioned in the introduction, twice a week my mother goes to "aerobics." This word means that old people are seeking to be younger in their exercise habits. It would be dangerous for elderly people, some of whom are unsteady on their feet, to jump around doing the kind of aerobics that young people do. So they sit in chairs. While seated, they exercise every muscle group in their bodies, making them feel invigorated. Aerobics reduce the risk of falls and hip fractures.

With a related purpose, scholars from Yale University come into my mother's facility to teach new ideas, providing aerobics for her mind, making her mind younger and healthier, and reducing the risk of Alzheimer's disease. Mayo Okada also attends some of these lectures. The active lives of my mother and Ms. Okada are examples of why Kenneth Manton finds decreasing rates of disability among the elderly.

Figure 7 shows the trend toward stronger old people. The bars show that, as they age, more and more people have trouble lifting a bag of groceries. For a moment, focus on the white vertical bars and ignore the black bars. The left-hand white bar shows that 17 percent of people ages 50 to 64 have trouble lifting a bag of groceries. In the next age bracket, ages 65 to 79, 31 percent of them have trouble lifting a bag of groceries. Thus, as you age, you are more likely to have trouble lifting heavy things. But when you compare the white bars to the black bars, you get an entirely different picture. The black bars in figure 7 show that nine years later, for each age group, people have less trouble lifting a bag of groceries. For example, comparing the central white and black bars, we see that for people ages 65 to 79, the percentage who have trouble lifting a bag of groceries declined from 31 percent to 25 percent in just nine years! At any specific age, old people are stronger than they used to be. Older people are developing stronger muscles than they used to have.[33]

Figure 7

Trouble Lifting a Bag of Groceries

(trends by age)

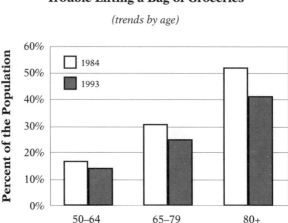

Data from Vicki Freedman and Linda Martin, "Understanding Trends in Functional Limitations among Older Americans," *American Journal of Public Health* 88, no. 10 (1998): 1457–62, table 3, p. 1461

Case History: Gordon Lewis

My friend Gordon Lewis has suffered from asthma since infancy. He is a Christian theologian who lives in Littleton, a suburb of Denver, Colorado. For years the doctors treated Gordon with prednisone, but it had adverse side effects, causing osteoporosis to such an extent that his spine became too calcium depleted to support his weight. Some of his vertebral bodies compressed, crushed. For months he suffered from several painful vertebral fractures, and for a time the combination of pain medicines and prednisone affected his ability to teach at Denver Seminary and write with clarity. He was writing his systematic theology (*Integrative Theology*), and the mental fog delayed for years his completion of the third volume.

One day Gordon nearly died. Blood clots built up in his legs because he had been inactive due to pain. The clots traveled to his lungs (pulmonary emboli), and he came within a hair's breadth of death in the intensive care unit.

Gordon's doctor referred him for cardiopulmonary rehabilitation. He was required to exercise as much as possible, while therapists monitored his heart rate and the state of his lungs. They taught him to take two deep breaths then exhale slowly through pursed lips. This kind of breathing was relaxing. Weight lifting not only strengthened his lungs, but also improved bone density.

He found this training so valuable that when the therapy program ended, he continued exercising. Two or three times a week he went to a local fitness center, warming up on a treadmill to get his pulse rate over one hundred, then "pumping iron" to exert all the major muscle groups of his body. A pulse rate of one hundred may seem to be a modest goal, until you consider that this was a seventy-six-year-old man with only 50 percent lung capacity. He said the weight lifting and deep breathing combined with meditation on biblical passages and great Christian truths allowed him to feel vigorous and energized.

A regular program of exercise allowed him to get off prednisone. The physician now treats him with antibiotics and prednisone only when he gets a respiratory infection. For two of the last three winters he has been free of bronchitis and has not had to use those medicines.

After Gordon's first wife of fifty-one years died, he decided to consult a Ph.D. in nutrition. He began eating health foods and dietary supplements. His second wife, Willa, has long been a health food fan. They avoid sweets and white processed flour, while emphasizing vegetables, fruit, turkey, and fish. Most of their groceries come from a health food store.

At seventy-six, Gordon is active—teaching one course a semester at Denver Seminary, speaking occasionally, and writing articles for publication. "I even preached at Breckenridge last summer," says Gordon. "That is a ski resort at over ten thousand feet elevation. Even though the air pressure is much less, I had no trouble breathing," he rejoices.

Gordon's ability to speak at Breckenridge shows the extent to which exercise, deep breathing, and a healthful diet have benefited him over the past decade. Again, this demonstrates why Kenneth Manton finds a decrease in disability among the elderly.

Strategy Eight: Exercise as Much as You Can

Exercise is one of the cornerstones of health. The irony about it is that young people and healthy people exercise, but others who could really reap the benefits of exercise (older people and sick people) are often couch potatoes. Like most physicians, I recommend walking every day as the most practical and sustainable form of exercise. I walk with my dog, K.C., every morning at dawn. A year ago my wife, Maureen O'Brien, joined us, which makes these walks a double pleasure.

The eighth strategy that I teach for managing your chronic disease is to exercise as much as you are able. The health benefits of exercise are extensive. For example, in my field, psychiatry, exercise has been shown to be as powerful as medications for treating (and preventing) major depression and anxiety disorders. It prevents Alzheimer's disease also.[34] Exercise leads to longer life. It prevents and/or treats a variety of chronic illnesses such as congestive heart failure, heart attacks, cancer, diabetes, and obesity. The antidepressant effects of exercise last longer than those of antidepressant medicines.[35]

I treat many patients for anxiety or depression, and I spend years suggesting that exercise would be a good idea. Most of them would rather take pills, sit on the sofa, and avoid exercise. Occasionally someone will begin walking and is usually astonished with how much better she or he feels.

Which News Is Dominant?

This chapter has focused on different aspects of the epidemic of chronic illness. In the first part of the chapter I talked about the bad news that there is an invisible epidemic and it is getting worse over the decades. In the second part I discussed the good news, namely that disability rates are falling among the elderly. We come now to the big question: Which is dominant, the bad or good news?

My own summary of the situation is that there is a mixture of bad and good news. But not everyone agrees. Some experts think I am too pessimistic. They think the good news eclipses or erases the bad.

How much optimism is warranted because of these falling disability rates among the elderly?[36] Clearly it is good news, but is it good news of sufficient magnitude to think that it is the dominant thing happening in health today? Should we ignore evidence of the epidemic, simply refuse to think about that information? Some experts say yes.

As you recall from the introduction, I am prone to major depression, and with this illness comes a tendency toward pessimism. Therefore I am vulnerable to self-doubt when other experts tell me I am too pessimistic. I am aware that I have a flaw in my ability to be realistic, such that I need to be vigilant in guarding against exaggerated pessimism. I don't believe I've been too pessimistic in this book, but I need to let you, my readers, decide. I will set before you the debate between the other experts and me, so that you can judge for yourselves whether the other experts are correct in thinking that things are rosier than the picture I have painted.

Experts Who Say I Am Too Pessimistic

James Fries proposes a theory called "compression of morbidity" that contradicts my point of view to some extent. Fries, a leading physician at the Stanford University School of Medicine, has been writing for twenty-five years in leading medical journals about his theory, and he has a lot of influence inside the medical profession. Fries proposes that there is progressively less sickness (morbidity) in society. As people get older, the age of onset of chronic disease and disability gets older at an even faster rate, so that old people spend fewer years being sick. This is what he means by morbidity being compressed. To say that morbidity is compressed means that there is progressively less time between the age of onset of disease and the age of death.

Is there evidence supporting Fries's theory? Yes, the data on declining rates of disability among the elderly support it. Fries says that disability rates have been declining among the elderly at about 2 percent per year, whereas mortality rates have been declining at 1 percent per year. The net result is a decrease in the total number of elderly disabled people. This is the primary evidence supporting Fries's theory of compression of morbidity. We have little information saying that the age of onset of chronic diseases has increased. In other words, Fries may have demonstrated a *compression of disability* among the elderly but has not proved a *compression of morbidity* (illness). Fries jumps to the conclusion that there is *no* epidemic of chronic illness. Instead, the population is getting more and more healthy.[37]

You might wonder how Fries reconciles his theory that there is progressively less chronic illness with the information I've cited showing the caribou effect, an increasing amount of chronic illness, and increasing rates of disability among working-age people and youths (figure 1). I asked him that by email.

Fries replied, "Point prevalence studies don't prove anything. 'Ain't it awful' studies are traditionally exaggerated, and nobody was sure about morbidity compression happening until 2002 anyway, so data from the early 1990s can't be used."[38]

In other words, Fries denies that there is an epidemic, primarily because he says that no studies before 2002 can be trusted. What happened in 2002? That was the year when two articles appeared in the *Journal of the American Medical Association*, showing that there is a decline in disability among the elderly.[39]

Fries continues in his email, "Gruenberg was right about expansion of morbidity through the mid 1970s, as acute diseases were being exchanged for chronic."[40] In other words, Fries thinks there was an epidemic of chronic illness at the time of Ernie Gruenberg's classic paper about the caribou effect. But by the 1990s the epidemic was over, Fries claims, replaced by a diminishing amount of illness. Of course, if Fries were correct, then the cost of healthcare should be going down.

In summary, from Fries's viewpoint, his theory of morbidity compression in the United States is an established fact. It is not just a theory but has been proved. For his theory *the* central proof is the declining rate of disability among the elderly, which was discovered by Kenneth Manton.[41] Rising rates of disability among youth and working-age people are irrelevant, according to Fries's theory, since his theory focuses only on what happens in the last decade or so of life.

I discussed Fries's view with an expert on disability, Stephen Kaye, who is head of research at the University of California San Francisco's Disability Statistics Center. He said, "I suspect there's some truth in Fries's compression of morbidity theory, at least for certain conditions. For example, the well observed decline in cardiovascular mortality over the past several decades seems to have been accompanied by a decline in disability due to cardiovascular conditions, so there's probably not only less mortality due to heart disease but also less illness and disability.

"I think the whole picture is more complicated, though," Kaye continues. "Recent data from the National Health Interview Survey show that among working-age adults with disabilities, the reported duration of the disabling condition (years since onset) has actually increased substantially from 1997 to 2002—a case of expansion rather than compression of morbidity."[42]

I also discussed these issues with Kenneth Manton, whose research on the elderly was the fountainhead and source from which all this optimism flowed. Professor Manton is at Duke University, where he teaches demography. I pointed out that research indicated there was an increasing amount of chronic illness among the elderly in the United States. Manton's response to me was that the decreasing rates of disability among the elderly proved that we were able to diagnose these illnesses earlier and manage them better, so they don't become disabilities.

Other Opinions

What do experts other than Fries, Kaye, and Manton think about this debate? The medical world is divided into different camps that don't communicate with one another much. Many physicians agree with Fries's idea that Americans are getting progressively healthier over the decades. Policy makers (such as government officials, insurance company executives, and hospital administrators) tend to believe the Partnership for Solution data that show Americans are getting progressively sicker over the decades. The astonishing thing is that almost no one realizes there is a debate, because the different parties neither talk to nor listen to one another.

There is even a debate about how to study the problem. Epidemiologists habitually modify their trend data using a technique called age-adjustment, which means that the impact of the aging of the population is hidden from public view. The reason we epidemiologists do that is because we assume everyone knows that aging causes increases in the rates of chronic illness, and age is such a powerful factor that it must be removed before anything else in the data becomes visible. It's like having to take the mud out of muddy water if you want to see what else is in the water. But, if what you want to study is reality (muddy water) instead of an epidemiologist's cleaned-up picture of reality, then you should not age-adjust the data, because the phenomenon of interest is precisely the impact of the aging of the population. Those who believe that the American people are getting healthier and healthier (Kenneth Manton and James Fries) present age-adjusted data, which makes things look unrealistically optimistic. After all, if the aging of the population is the primary reason there is an epidemic, and if they use age-adjustment to artificially remove that factor from their data, of course they are not going to find an epidemic! If scholars like Manton and Fries do use age-adjustment, they should publish a disclaimer that says, "Because we age-adjusted the data, we cannot make any comments about whether or not there is an epidemic of chronic illness."

Are You Confused?

Some readers tell me they are confused. Am I saying that people are healthier and healthier or that they are sicker and sicker? The answer is that I am proposing a paradox that both things could be happening simultaneously. If we define "healthier" to mean having an improved quality of life, and if we define "sick" to mean carrying a medical diagnosis, then it is possible for both things to be happening simultaneously. A larger and larger proportion of the population could carry a long-term diagnosis but have a quality of life that is better than it used to be. These trends are especially evident among the elderly.

Earlier I mentioned the media message that is promoted by health-care opinion leaders, namely that "people are getting healthier and healthier because of breakthroughs in medicine." And they are, if you mean they are living longer with diseases that might have been lethal only a few short years ago. In everyday terminology it also means that these *healthy* people are taking more medications, requiring more medical procedures, and must see more than one doctor to maintain their level of health. They are living longer, healthier lives with a chronic illness. For most of us, *health* means feeling good. Many of the chronically ill do not feel good and would not consider themselves healthy. Yet advances in medical science make it possible for them to go on living and enjoying to a certain extent what life has to offer. And for this they are grateful and even joyous. But they wouldn't necessarily describe themselves as *healthy*.

The medical media message is a large part of what is making this chapter so confusing. James Fries's theory of compression of morbidity supports that media message, which in turn supports the multibillion-dollar infrastructure of research and development as seen in pharmaceutical companies, genetics engineering companies, and American medical schools. James Fries's theory is well-known among physicians. Catherine Hoffman's and Gerard Anderson's data are largely ignored because the idea of an epidemic of chronic illness affecting half the population would be difficult to reconcile with that media message.

I don't think that the decreasing rate of disability among the elderly (the Kenneth Manton data) is evidence that we should forget the epidemic of chronic illness. A diagnosis of chronic illness is different from the level of disability. The two variables are independent of one another. I concede that James Fries may have proved that there is a *compression of disability* among the elderly, in the sense that I might become disabled at age eighty instead of age sixty. But I reject Fries's claim to have proved a *compression of morbidity* (that there is less chronic illness). I reject it because Catherine Hoffman and Gerard Anderson have shown there is an epidemic increase in the prevalence of chronic illness and the prevalence of comorbidity among the elderly.

These debates are not the central focus of this book. I told you about them because it is my responsibility to inform you that these issues are controversial and that my viewpoint is more pessimistic than Fries's view. The summary of the difference is this: Other experts look at the declining rate of disability among the elderly and are wildly optimistic, whereas I prefer a mixed picture—appreciating the declining rate among the elderly but not forgetting the climbing rate of chronic illnesses among people of every age group.

5

THE VALUE OF
SPIRITUAL RESOURCES

Chronic diseases are usually incurable, but I have introduced eight strategies with which people have managed to live acceptable lives despite having such diseases. In the remainder of this book I present twelve more strategies for living with chronic illness.

Strategy Nine: Use Spiritual Coping

As the problem of paying for medical care gets worse, many people are worried. They are beginning to give up on traditional methods of struggling with chronic illness and are turning to spiritual approaches.

When I was in medical school between 1972 and 1976, religion was considered irrelevant to health. During my medical career, however, there has been a revolution in thinking within the medical community. Current medical research indicates that religious coping (which in the medical vocabulary is called spiritual coping) increases people's resilience in many ways. In this chapter you will read four colorful case histories that illustrate strategy nine, which is to use spiritual coping. But first we have to briefly review why medical researchers say that spirituality is important, so that you can understand what I'm driving at with these four case histories.

Spiritual coping can improve your health in a variety of ways.

- It increases your community involvement and social network (strategy one), because you are likely to belong to a congregation or prayer group.
- It provides a coherent meaning and purpose that makes sense out of the chaos of illness.[1]
- It tends to decrease your risk-taking behaviors.[2]
- It increases your altruism so that you focus on others rather than yourself.[3]
- The liturgical calendar and discipline of weekly prayer and worship tend to force you to withdraw from the bombardment of everyday life on a regular schedule, thereby reducing your exposure to unremitting stress.[4]

All five of these factors have an impact on health, and spirituality has an impact on all five factors. In a dynamic and evolving field of medical research, these are among the issues that are under investigation today.

Some readers ask whether current medical research shows that all religions promote health equally, or are the adherents of certain world religions healthier than adherents of others. There are two answers. First, almost zero research has been done comparing the health effects of one religion versus another, so the question cannot be answered. When medical researchers speak as if all forms of spirituality are equally valid, they are making an assumption not based on empirical data. This assumption comes from two sources—the American idea that pluralism is good and the medical orientation that our treatments should be available to all patients, regardless of race, gender, creed, color, or religion. Because of these ideas, it is unlikely that you will see research funded in the United States that compares the different world religions in a horse race, and if such research ever were done, it is unlikely that it would be published in leading medical journals, and if it were published, it would not be believed because people would suspect that the study was motivated by some covert apologetic purpose.

Second, most of the published medical research on spirituality has been done on Christian forms of spirituality. Usually these research reports appear in the medical journals reporting a positive effect of "spirituality" in general, ignoring the question of whether what is true of Christian spirituality can be generalized to other forms of spirituality.

My overall goal in this chapter is to show how spirituality enables people to deal with chronic diseases. Other goals are to understand what the term *spiritual coping* means when it appears in medical research journals and to gain an appreciation for the spiritual pluralism of America.

Negative Spiritual Coping

Although spiritual coping has an impact on health, the impact is not always positive. Kenneth Pargament, one of the leaders in this field, writes: "Spirituality has a darker side. For a small but significant number of people, illness can trigger spiritual struggles. These struggles take the form of anger at God, feeling punished for one's transgressions, believing that the illness is the work of the devil, feeling abandoned by God, or religious conflict with dogma, congregation members and clergy. Spiritual struggles, when unresolved, have been linked to depression, poorer quality of life, poorer self-rated health, slower recovery, and greater risk of mortality among the medically ill."[5]

How does unhealthy differ from healthy spirituality? The most carefully designed study asked six hundred hospitalized sick people about their faith, beliefs, and spiritual experiences, then followed them for two years to determine who died and who survived. Working backward, the researchers determined what kind of spirituality at the beginning increased the probability of death within the next two years. They found that those who thought the devil was responsible for their suffering were more likely to die than those who didn't think that way. Also those who wondered whether God had abandoned them had an increased probability of death. Ditto for those who questioned whether God loved them.[6] Apparently religious turmoil is toxic. On average, however, spiritual coping improves a person's health.

If the reader wants to learn more about medical research on religious coping, a good place to start is with Dr. Harold Koenig's book *The Healing Power of Faith*. See also Koenig's discussion in *JAMA* of an eighty-three-year-old woman who uses faith to cope with persistent, severe pain.[7]

Positive Spiritual Coping

In a pluralistic world, the word *spirituality* has different meanings.[8] The next four case histories will provide different perspectives on what the phrase "spiritual coping" can mean. At the end of this chapter you will discover that, despite the differences in their spiritual coping, there are unifying themes in these four case histories.

DONNA JOBLONICKY

Donna Joblonicky of Spring Hill, Florida, describes herself as a spiritual person, though it is a different spirituality than she experienced in the Catholic Church as a youngster. A close encounter with death at age forty-seven, four years ago, has shaped her spiritually.

As a teenager, Donna lost interest in church ceremonies and stopped going to church. She was neither religious nor spiritual prior to the crisis in her mid-forties, when her ulcerative colitis flared up for an entire year. She could hardly get out of the bathroom and suffered almost continuous pain and bleeding. Exhausted, she finally consented to surgery to remove her entire large intestine. It was major-league surgery, lasting seven hours. Her husband, Bruce, still shudders at the memory of the surgeon saying, "She could have died!" The pathologist found Donna's large intestine was in tatters, on the brink of disintegration. Donna had not realized she was so sick, skating on thin ice for the year prior to the surgery. Looking back on the experience, she understands that she came very close to dying. Now, with proper care, Donna's disease can be managed.

Since Donna's surgery, she has been spiritual. She prays every morning for guidance and has a continual sense of comfort from spirituality. She doesn't go to church. Whether her spirituality has to do with God or with some benevolent energy or power, she doesn't know.

She says that her prayers are pleadings for immediate, practical help. If she's having a bad day, she will shoot off a prayer for a parking space. The next thing you know a parking space is available next to her place of work, and she says to her higher power, "Okay, I know you're there taking care of me!" She has a sense of being affirmed the way a child is comforted knowing its mother is nearby.

Prior to the surgery Donna felt a need to be in control of every aspect of her life. Since her surgery she has been relinquishing control to her spirituality. For her this means learning to trust that things are going to work out, even if they go in a different direction than she wanted.

"I have a lot of conversations with my spirituality," she says. "I grew up in a very structured Catholic church, but what I have now is different. It is gentle and comforting, something new and unexpected in my life. I belong to a prayer chain. My friends and I keep one another in our thoughts as we go through the day, which is also comforting." This is an example of how spirituality can increase your social network (strategy one).

Donna has lupus, but it has subsided, and her joint pain has finally settled down. Because of the prednisone that she has taken for the last fifteen years, she has osteoporosis. The bones in her feet are fragile and have broken three times. Because of this, Donna scoots around nursing homes in an electric wheelchair on the job as a nurse practitioner. But Donna doesn't feel sorry for herself. Like her father before her, she is a go-getter who keeps her chin up when she's afflicted, determined to continue working and carrying on.

"Every day I am grateful that I wake up in a warm bed with my husband," Donna continues. "So many people live with severe poverty. They don't have enough to eat, or their diseases are worse than mine. Here we are in a wonderful home with heat and running water. We have nice vehicles and go out to restaurants to eat. I am almost always thankful for how nice our life is. This is another aspect of my spirituality. Life is a gift!

"When something bad happens," Donna says, "I try to look for the positive in the situation, try to find a lesson in it so I don't have to go through it again. I teach my patients the same thing, if possible. 'Okay,' I say, 'so this is the negative part of your life, but let's remember the positive things in your life, like how your marriage was before you lost your husband.' It is almost an imaging thing that I teach in the nursing homes, helping people remember the blessings of life. I am very interested in alternative methods of healing.

"The nursing homes I go to are so different from hospitals," she says. "In a hospital everyone is so rushed and frustrated! Even in medical offices the doctors and nurses are harried, trying to see fifty patients a day, one every ten minutes. The pace is slower in nursing homes. People are friendlier. It's like one big family. People care about one another. If I'm having a bad day, people will notice and give me an extra hug. That helps a lot. It is part of the spiritual comfort that I live with.

"I have a philosophy of trying to get away from people who are unhealthy," Donna says. "My first two marriages were difficult. I got divorced because of difficult or bad relationships. I met my third husband, Bruce, through a dating service. He's great! He and I are on the same wavelength to such an extent that we are often thinking the same thing without having talked about it in advance. Bruce is very attentive to my needs, like saying that we should stop at McDonald's on the highway because he knows that I may need to use the bathroom. I have such a supportive marriage this time!"

As I said, Donna considers herself spiritual but she isn't sure that there is a God. She believes that there is an energy or life force that helps and guides her and that everything spiritual is positive. Personally I am not ready to trust anything and everything spiritual, because I've been impressed with what the apostle John writes in the New Testament:

> Dear friends, do not believe every spirit, but test the spirits to see whether they are from God, because many false prophets have gone out into the world. This is how you can recognize the Spirit of God: Every spirit that acknowledges that Jesus Christ has come in the flesh is from God, but every spirit that does not acknowledge Jesus is not from God. This is the spirit of the antichrist, which you have heard is coming and even now is already in the world.
>
> 1 John 4:1–3

Donna Joblonicky's spiritual coping is not anchored in any particular religion. She has a homemade recipe of ideas and experiences relating to her perception of a life force. Her ideas are idiosyncratic, but many medical people would think that she provides an excellent example of what the phrase *spiritual coping* means.

Morris Days

We turn now to a man who uses a traditional form of spiritual coping as he wrestles with chronic illness. Morris Days's spirituality has made it possible for him to endure the physical suffering he's been through. Were it not for faith, he would not have made it. Because of his spirituality Morris, of Reston, Virginia, feels that life is good and that he is blessed as he awaits a lung transplant, even though he is not sure whether or not he will live another year.

"Verily," he says, "with every difficulty there is relief. Remaining in the Lord has given me the urge to get better. With greater illness has come greater faith and trust in the Lord."

Morris was brought up in Philadelphia in the days when African Americans didn't have many opportunities because of segregation. Morris's mother was serious about religion and took him to a Baptist church, where they both sang in the choir.

As he grew up, Morris got involved in the Civil Rights Movement. Malcolm X and the Black Muslims influenced him as well. After serving in the Army, Morris worked at a variety of jobs and didn't go to college until late in life, at which time he studied criminal justice in Philadelphia, hoping to be a parole officer. Eventually, at thirty-six, he went to Temple University Law School. As a lawyer he worked first in criminal defense law in Philadelphia then in telecommunications law in Tyson's Corner, Virginia. Prior to his illness he was busy with traveling and speaking.

At forty-one Morris had some pains in his stomach. An X-ray revealed an enlarged spleen. This was removed surgically and discovered to be full of non-Hodgkin's lymphoma. Aggressive chemotherapy cured the cancer over the next two years. But then other things went wrong. The operation to remove his spleen left him with scar tissue inside his abdomen, which turned into a nightmare worse than the cancer, namely bowel obstruction due to adhesions. He had nine abdominal surgeries, some of them gruesome. Only his faith allowed Morris to hang onto his sanity.

"The Lord is merciful," says Morris. "At first I didn't see it. But eventually I realized that he allowed the cancer to be diagnosed at an early enough time so that it could be treated. He only gave me one thing at a time, so that I wouldn't be overwhelmed. The chemotherapy ended before the bowel obstructions began."

Meanwhile Morris got short of breath because of scarring of his lungs. There is no proof what caused it, but the theory is that chemotherapy damaged his lungs. Today he needs a constant flow of oxygen to survive. Without a lung transplant soon, he won't survive even with oxygen. Fortunately the chances of getting a new lung in the next year are good.

Every day Morris reads the Koran and prays with his second wife, Aisha. He spends two hours a day at the mosque, volunteering to help immigrant Muslims from Pakistan, Somalia, Afghanistan, and Sudan figure out how to solve practical problems. As a disabled volunteer, he practices for free what he calls public interest law. For example, Muslims from these other countries are afraid of the government because of the tyranny they lived under back in the motherland. They are proud and don't want charity. Morris counsels them that they might consider applying for services from the local governments inside the United States to help the senior citizens in their families. He helps them fill out application forms, counsels them about immigration law, and advises them how to fight discrimination.

He has only enough energy to be active four hours a day. So he returns home after two hours and fields phone calls from his apartment in a subsidized housing complex for disabled people.

I asked Morris what he thinks of Osama bin Laden and al Qaeda. He gave me a reply similar to that of Shiqirije Krosi in the last chapter.

"Al Qaeda is terrible!" Morris says. "They are the opposite of Islam. It is atrocious that they perpetuate violence for religious motives. What they are doing is not allowed in Islam. The Koran does not allow or ordain killing innocent people and children. There is nothing in the Koran about spreading Islam through terrorism. Historically there has always been religious freedom in Islamic countries, freedom to practice other religions. Islam has always had an attitude of brotherhood with other faiths."

The following table shows where Islam stands among the major spiritual traditions of the world. Islam is the second most popular spirituality in the world, after Christianity. Islam is growing faster than Christianity, partly because of a high birth rate. The third and fourth largest spiritualities in the world are Hinduism and Buddhism respectively.[9]

Table 2

Major Spiritual Traditions in the World and in the United States

(in millions of people)

	World		United States	
	Millions of People	**Percent of the Population**	**Millions of People**	**Percent of the Population**
Christian	2,000	33%	239	84%
Islamic	1,186	20%	4	1%
Hindu	804	13%	1	less than 1%
Buddhist	364	6%	3	1%
Jewish	15	less than 1%	6	2%
None of the Above	1,687	28%	30	11%
Total	6,056	100%	283	100%

The bottom row shows that there are six billion people in the world (6,056 million). Of these, two billion, or one-third (33 percent) say they are Christian, as shown in the top row, middle column. The second row, middle column shows that one billion, or one-fifth (20 percent) of the world's population say they are Muslim. Other religions are less popular than these two.

To Morris the Koran makes more sense than the Bible, so he converted from Christianity to Islam. He says the Koran explains the same Bible stories he learned as a child, but makes them more clear and understandable. Some things in the Bible make no sense to Morris, like why God would get tired and need a rest on the seventh day, after making the heavens and the earth. Morris says that Allah holds you responsible for your actions, unlike Christianity which tends to let people off the hook because Jesus died for their sins. For Morris the bottom-line issue is that Islam makes more sense of the world than Christianity. When Morris prays as a Muslim, he has more of a feeling of personal and direct access to God than when he prayed as a Christian. Islamic prayers, which are in Arabic, are soothing to the ear and when they are translated into English, the words make a lot of sense, he says. Allah, the creator of the heavens and the earth, is directly available through prayer. Morris's experience of Allah is immediate and interactive, which Morris likes very much.

He belongs to the All Dulles Area Muslim Society, which is a large, mainstream Sunni mosque in Herndon, Virginia. He is a mainstream Muslim, which means that he follows exactly what the Prophet Mohammad prescribed 1,423 years ago, as opposed to the Nation of Islam (also known as the Black Muslims).

How has spirituality allowed Morris to remain upbeat as he lives with chronic illness? He tells me that his religion has transformed him. He now accepts the inevitability of death and is not afraid. He accepts his disabilities and the life he now lives. "I hope that Allah allows me to die when I am serving him the best," Morris says, "like when I am performing a charity or worshipping. I used to be afraid of death. But now my deepest wish is that when I die, I do so as a good Muslim."

When he had cancer, a visualization nurse asked Morris and other cancer patients to imagine the immune cells of their bodies battling against and winning the war against the cancer cells. She said, "Use anything that works for you."

"I imagined the cells of my body fighting with the power of Allah against cancer cells," Morris says. "After all, among all the millions of sperm cells that had a chance to fertilize the egg when I was conceived, Allah chose one particular sperm cell and empowered it to be the one predestined to become me. Similarly it is possible to visualize the immune system of my body, empowered by Allah, fighting for 'me' against the cancer cells that are 'not me.'"

Morris was reluctant to talk with me about his experience of the supernatural, but because he trusted me, he shared the following story. When his abdomen was not healing after the worst of the bowel surgeries, he despaired for his life. He thought of the prayer that Jonah said when enclosed in the belly of a whale. Because of not performing his duties, Jonah had been swallowed by a whale, according to the Koran. Jonah was inside the darkness of the whale, inside the darkness of the ocean, and the whale dove to the bottom of the sea, so there was triple darkness. There Jonah cried to Allah, saying, "You alone can save me from this calamity." When Morris repeated the prayer of Jonah, his abdominal wound began to heal, and in three days he was able to leave the hospital. He considers it a miracle.

Today Morris faces a lung transplant knowing that whatever happens, it will be okay because he is in Allah's hands, whether he lives or dies. There are many things to be afraid of in the days ahead. If Morris didn't have faith, he could be overwhelmed with terror. He will have to endure the discomfort of being on a respirator and the risk that his tissue and that of the transplanted lung will not be compatible. There is always a chance that the medicine used to prevent rejection of the new lung will weaken Morris's immune system so that the cancer comes back. Only because of his trust in Allah can Morris relax.

"If the surgery doesn't go well," Morris says, "or I don't survive the surgery, I have no complaints. I've had a nice life. I have a wonderful wife and a nice apartment. I am not wealthy, trying to live on disability income. But I feel okay with myself, and this is all because of my religion.

"In the Koran, when Mohammad was facing hardship, Allah said to him, 'Have we not expanded for you your breast and removed from you the burden that almost broke your back?' This meant that Allah allowed Mohammad to feel better ('expanded your breast') and supported Mohammad. It means, 'Verily, with every difficulty there is relief.' I say that a lot when I'm not feeling well. It reminds me to count my blessings. It's a very good feeling I get from my religion. For the last nine years Allah has been so real to me that it is almost frightening.

"When I was in the cancer ward," Morris continues, "some patients didn't go home. I met a nine-year-old boy in the game room, where they had a TV and Play Station. He was a Hispanic boy with a swollen face. He said that if he died, he would ask God to help me get better. He was not a Muslim and didn't know I was a Muslim. That boy died a few days later, whereas I walked out of the hospital and got better.

"So now I am spending my energy paying back," says Morris. "I am not paying back Allah, because Allah doesn't need anything from me. I am paying back humanity by helping people. I am sharing my gratitude.

"I've never been to Mecca," he says. "My fondest dream would be, if I get a good lung transplant, to make a hajj. But if I can't go to Mecca because I am still too sick, I would want my wife to go without me."

At the end of our conversation Morris said a prayer in Arabic. Then he translated it: "May the peace, mercy, and blessings of Allah be upon you, Dr. Boyd."

REVEREND KOSHU

In this book, as we observe how people find deliverance from suffering, it is inevitable that we would cross paths with a man whose life work was focused on understanding why we suffer and seeking deliverance from suffering, namely Siddhartha Gautama, who lived from 566 to 486 B.C. in Nepal. He investigated this question long before me. At age thirty-five he became the Buddha, the third most famous person to ever live on earth (after Jesus and Mohammad). In New England where I live and work, the Buddha's philosophy is becoming more and more influential in medical settings.

Jim Koshu, a Buddhist, can help us understand spiritual coping from a Buddhist's perspective. Jim grew up a nice Catholic kid, a gymnast who loved to tumble and had a tendency to be hot tempered. If he hadn't liked girls so much, he might have become a Catholic priest. After high school he married a Methodist girl named Nanci, to whom he has been married for thirty-seven years. Nanci was pregnant when Jim was drafted and sent to fight the war in Vietnam. He ended up in the 101st Airborne Division and went to language school to learn Vietnamese. He served in Vietnam from 1967 to 1968, where he interrogated Viet Cong soldiers, because he spoke the language. In the process, he discovered that the fight against Communism had little to do with the war in South Vietnam. It was, he told me, a religious war. This was news to me.

Vietnam was part of the French colonial empire. Jim said that the French imposed Catholicism on the populace that was 80 percent Buddhist. Even when the French pulled out and American troops moved in to prop up the South Vietnamese government, Jim said that a South Vietnamese citizen had to be Catholic to vote, own land, or hold a government office. The government was anti-Buddhist. There was a law that no more than five Buddhists could gather in a temple at any one time. Jim came to see the Vietnam War as a war against the Buddhist majority.

Because he spoke the language, Jim believed he understood what the Vietnamese were telling him about the war and that other American troops were ignorant, believing incorrectly that it was a war against Communism. After a while Jim felt guilty about the killing he had done as a soldier. He sought the counsel of a Catholic army chaplain.

The chaplain said, "Don't let it bother you. They're just animals!" At that instant Jim lost his Christian faith. He understood the priest's use of the word *animals* to mean that the Vietnamese were heathen, not converted to Catholicism. This dovetailed with how Jim thought about the war, that it was a war of Catholics using the sword to beat the Buddhist majority into submission.

In Saigon he went into a Buddhist temple that was part of the Thich Nhat Hanh sect. This is the same Thich Nhat Hanh who, three decades later, became the second most influential Buddhist teacher in the United States (second only to the Dalai Lama).[10] The monk taught peace. If one killed, one would have to deal with the karma of killing. This made sense to Jim.

"There is no excuse for war," Jim concluded.

The monk taught Jim five mindfulness trainings. The Buddha said it was wrong to kill, yet the monk claimed that the Buddha had killed someone. On a boat the Buddha once met a man who bragged about murdering five hundred women and children and promised to go on killing women and children. The Buddha pushed him overboard so he drowned. Then the Buddha had to deal with the negative karma that came from killing.

James Koshu became a Buddhist and remained one from that day on—for thirty-six years now. Eight years ago, as Jim's declining health forced him to retire from a career in law enforcement, he studied for the Buddhist priesthood under Master Taicho, of the Hongaku Jodo priesthood, and was ordained and given the name Koshu Dari, which means "Wholesome Attitude."

When Jim returned from the Vietnam War, thirty-six years ago, both his family and in-laws were appalled by his new religion. Both families said Nanci was a saint for sticking with him. Over three decades Jim and Nanci have learned to be accepting of each other's religion. Jim says his wife became something of a Buddhist kind of Christian, even though she still goes to a United Methodist church.

"I'm afraid to go to church with my wife," Jim laughs. "The roof might fall in!"

Today Reverend Koshu is an associate priest to the main Vietnamese temple in Buffalo, New York, the Chua Tu Hieu Temple. Reverend Koshu's webpage gives a clearer synopsis of Buddhism than anything else I've read (hometown.aol.com/reverendkoshu/index.htm). He spends much of his time counseling people of the South Vietnamese community of about two thousand people whom the American government relocated into the city of Buffalo.

What can we learn from Reverend Koshu about how to live with chronic illness? At age forty-four Jim had a heart attack and five-vessel bypass surgery. He developed Bell's palsy and a reaction to prednisone. He has had to contend with heart failure, a stroke, sleep apnea, and diabetes. Every day he takes five medicines (Glucophage, Accupril, atenolol, Celexa, and hydrochlorothiazide).

"Every time I turn around," he says, "something else seems to go wrong, but I am not much bothered by my ailments. About the only thing I regret is that I won't be able to kick the soccer ball around with my five-year-old grandson when he gets a little older. Other than that the illnesses don't have much impact on me. I meditate an hour a day, and when I do, I'm aware of the body's creaks and pains, like my legs falling asleep. The path for me is to learn to eliminate my craving for good health. Craving is the path to suffering. If I extinguish the desire for existence, then I will avoid the need to be reborn after I die. I view my illnesses like a bad dream. It is simply something that happened. I don't dwell on my illnesses. I simply walk away from them. For example," Jim continues, "I can't have sex with my wife anymore. I'm impotent, so I just walk away from it."

Impotence is common among people with chronic illnesses, but few men are gutsy enough to declare it in public. While some sick people are impotent, a larger number have zero libido or an aversion to sex engendered by discomfort during intercourse. I applaud Jim's courage in trying to help others by openly discussing this issue in a book that will be read by other sick people and their sexual partners.

"The impotence is because of my diseases," Jim continues. "The doctors at a V.A. hospital suggested an implant, which I thought was ridiculous, the idea of pumping the thing up! A guy like me can't take Viagra because it is dangerous if you have heart disease. My wife is real understanding. She says that after thirty-seven years she needs to give it a rest. She says that if the doctor recommends an implant again, she'll beat him up. She makes me laugh. Humor is one way that I live with the illnesses. So I just deal with the sexual impotence. I dismiss it. I had to practice detachment." (Jim's use of Buddhist detachment is not what I would recommend for readers of this book. There are other ways for a couple to have sexual intimacy without intercourse.)

Reverend Koshu's webpage quotes the Buddha as saying that the Noble Truth of Suffering is this: "Decay is suffering, illness is suffering, death is suffering. Presence of objects we hate is suffering, separation from objects we love is suffering, not to obtain what we desire is suffering." The cause of suffering is "thirst for pleasure, thirst for existence, thirst for prosperity."[11]

The Noble Truth of the Cessation of Suffering "is the complete cessation of this thirst—a cessation which consists in the absence of every passion with the abandoning of this thirst, with the doing away with it, with the deliverance from it, with the destruction of desire." How do you accomplish that? By means of the Eightfold Path.

"It's like when I lost my son, Todd," Jim tells me. "That was devastating for my wife. Nanci didn't know how I could handle it so well. I simply practiced detachment."

"How can you detach from someone you loved?" I ask. I was reminded of how devastated I was when my son Justin died. It took me years to recover.

"We Buddhists live in the present moment," Jim replies. "The past no longer exists, and the future doesn't exist yet. The present is all we have. When Todd was alive I loved him deeply. But when he died, I was able to let go without regrets. I'll always remember him and always love him. But I was able to detach from the need for him to be present. Eventually my wife came to see it that way. She learned slowly to detach, which is what I mean when I say Nanci is a little bit like a Buddhist, despite being a Christian.

"My body is a suit," Jim continues. "It is subject to wrinkles and the fabric tears. The mind, however, is a perpetually running thing, an energy. When we are reincarnated, it is like the continuity of electricity, which explains how two-year-old children can play Mozart. The task is to learn how to put that energy to rest, so that it is no longer thirsty for life."

Throughout the medical world in the United States pain management and stress management experts are promoting mindfulness (which is another name for Buddhism).[12] The most popular medical book on that subject is *Full Catastrophe Living*, by Jon Kabat-Zinn.[13]

I am impressed with how active Jim's life is. The afternoon I interviewed him he also conducted a funeral and counseled a friend whose husband was about to die. He is a pastoral care volunteer at the local hospital, assistant abbot with a Buddhist clergy group, and active in the antiwar movement. In addition, Jim is on the board of trustees of the New Mexico Institute of Buddhist Studies. He's a dynamo!

"I have to remain active," Jim says. "It keeps me from dwelling on my illnesses. If I just sit around, I get depressed about the state of the world. I feel better if I'm actively serving people." Jim's idea about keeping busy is strategy 16.

WALTER UNGER AND SPIRITUAL VIRTUES

The most popular form of spiritual coping in the world is Christianity. When I use the word *Christian*, I am referring simply to how people answer the question, "What is your religion?" There are many varieties of Christianity represented in this book. In this chapter I have room to discuss only one type, namely a Protestant variety. Catholic and Orthodox spiritual coping styles are represented elsewhere in the book. In the United States most of those who call themselves Christian are Protestant, but in the world as a whole, things are different. Half the Christians in the world are Roman Catholic, and Protestants are in the minority.[14]

Walter Unger was president of Columbia Bible College in Abbotsford, British Columbia (forty-five minutes east of Vancouver), and an accomplished hockey player. At age fifty-four he was playing hockey with some of the guys. Suddenly there was a breakaway opportunity. He grabbed the puck and should have been able to skate like greased lightning toward the goal, but, mysteriously, his feet barely moved. They felt like cement. Friends captured it all on videotape, that day when Walter blew it, when he was wide open and could not get mobilized.

That was the first sign that something was wrong. Walter shrugged it off.

A while later he was walking to work, an invigorating distance of two miles. He loved his job, had raised millions of dollars for Columbia, and enjoyed being commander-in-chief. That day, about halfway to school, he hit a wall of exhaustion. It was the most peculiar thing, to be limping and struggling for no good reason. It began to happen every day.

Walter went to a neurologist and told him his muscles were twitching and that he got exhausted walking to work. The neurologist shrugged it off, making a diagnosis of "benign fasciculation." No nerve conduction test was done, which in retrospect was a shame, because there was an outside chance that the disease might have responded to treatment had it been correctly diagnosed at that early stage.

Years passed. Walter's exhaustion and limping got worse. Whatever this mystery was, it was progressive. A different neurologist made a diagnosis of Lou Gehrig's disease. Of course, hearing this diagnosis was catastrophic. Fortunately, it was also wrong. Two months later the doctors changed their minds and said Walter had chronic inflammatory demyelinating polyneuropathy (CIDP). This is a cousin of Lou Gehrig's disease but milder. CIDP involves a progressive deterioration of the nerves, with pain and progressive paralysis starting in the feet. It is slower and less malignant than Lou Gehrig's disease. Muscles wither, however, and like Lou Gehrig's, there is no treatment.

Because of the disease, Walter retired earlier than planned from his position as president of Columbia Bible College. Today, at sixty-seven, Walter wears braces that hold up his feet, because his muscles are so wasted that his feet flap on the ground (called foot drop). There is pain later in the day, despite taking Neurontin. This autoimmune disease hobbles his gait. Walter is by nature competitive, athletic, and he likes to win, but today he cannot keep up with his wife, Laura, when she walks slowly. His legs are feeble. He needs a nap every afternoon.

At the Bible college, where he is president emeritus, he is admired and respected. He continues to have enough energy to do the things he loves, such as teaching and preaching. His arms are not affected at this early stage of the disease.

The worst part of CIDP is the ominous sense of progressive deterioration from which there is no rescue. Thus the future is shadowed
by storm clouds that have not yet reached into the present. The worst
part of the disease is neither the exhaustion nor the foot drop but
the pessimistic prognosis.

When I first phoned Walter to interview him, I could not reach
him. He and Laura were off on a Caribbean cruise. They have been
traveling as much as possible in recent years, because they want to
squeeze all the juice out of life before Walter is no longer able to go.
At the time of our interview, Walter was using neither crutches nor
wheelchair.

"I love the paper you gave at the Evangelical Theological Society
in Colorado Springs,"[15] Walter tells me. "I think you are right that the
issue with chronic illness is that we need to focus on the God-human
relationship, instead of focusing only on healing."

When I first proposed to interview Walter, he was humble and said
he wasn't coping very well with his disease and didn't think he had
much to say. That's the way Christians are. They figure they don't
have much to contribute. He agreed to the interview on the grounds
that it might be therapeutic for him, but he thought the interview
would be useless for me.

Like a pot of tea, Walter steeped over the course of a few days.
By the time we actually talked, he had a lot to say about spiritual
coping, which took me by surprise. I had expected to be talking to a
depressed man who felt defeated by his disease. That's what he led
me to expect in our previous conversation.

True, he is depressed and angry sometimes, but that passes and is
not the dominant characteristic of Walter's life. He had been reading over the paper I had written, and that set him to thinking more
optimistically about his illness.

"I refuse to be defined by this disease," Walter says. "I am not just
a case of CIDP! I want to be defined as a servant of Jesus Christ, a
man of God, and a teacher. The illness is peripheral, not central, to
my identity.

"I've learned many lessons from this experience," Walter continues. "Primarily I've learned humility. I have type A personality. I've
raised millions of dollars for this school. I am competitive and love
coming in first. But now I've come up against limitations that I can't

get around. I can no longer be the best and can't even keep up with Laura when we're walking! I've learned to accept my helplessness, because there is nothing I can do that will have any impact on the progression of this disease. We men like to do things to solve problems. Well, I've got an illness about which nothing can be done, a problem that has no solution. Being helpless engenders greater dependence on God. The harder my life gets, the more I learn to turn to the Lord for my strength.

"I've learned to accept my limitations, to adjust my lifestyle. Now I sit on a stool when I'm teaching a class of church history or theology."

"Does the illness cloud your ability to think?" I ask.

"Fortunately, no," he replies. "My mind has been spared. It is mostly that I have problems with my legs.

"I've also learned to be more sympathetic with people who are ill. The other day I ran into one of my old golf buddies. He's been diagnosed with cancer. Tomorrow I will visit him in the hospital. Because of my disease, I can be more compassionate. God is using the disease to teach me things. I like what you say in your paper, Jeff, that to find the purpose of a disease we need to look to the future instead of looking to the past. There is a *telos* to illness, a purpose that God has in mind for our sanctification, and it has to do with learning spiritual virtues."

In that paper on the theology of chronic illness, I said that a disease may appear random, destructive, and pointless if we consider only the past, but it has a future-oriented purpose, namely to teach us spiritual virtues. We say, "Things happen for a reason," but we need to remember that in all probability the reason lies in the future not in the past. When a boy is born blind, this is what Jesus says. The reason is in the future not in the past (John 9:1–3).

I also said that all this emphasis on faith healing in the Christian church today is different than what the Church Fathers talked about. They talked about illness but rarely mentioned faith healing. Most of them "agree that suffering, even from disease, when it afflicts the Christian is sent or permitted for his ultimate good by a God who loves him and will cause all things to work together for his good."[16] This concept comes from Romans 8:28. Augustine and other Fathers cite Hebrews 12:6: "the Lord disciplines those he loves, and he punishes everyone he accepts as a son."[17] In other words, the Fathers advised us to accept unavoidable adversity as an opportunity to learn from God lessons that we might otherwise not want to learn. The "lessons" are about spiritual virtues.[18]

A virtue is something excellent about a person that leads him or her to live well. Virtues are good habits. Plato and Aristotle speak of virtues that concern a person's moral character. Wisdom (meaning insight and good judgment), courage (bravery), self-restraint (moderation or temperance), and ethics (justice) are virtues discussed by the Greek philosophers. The New Testament adds three spiritual virtues: faith, hope, and love.

According to the New Testament, your spiritual life consists of personal growth in the direction of becoming more like Jesus Christ (Rom. 13:14). The spiritual virtues are lifestyle qualities that describe how your personality changes as you make that journey.

Along these lines, Walter Unger says, "My disease can bring me into greater conformity with Christ. We live in a fallen world," Walter continues. "Francis Schaeffer, in his book *The God Who Is There*, writes about the results of the fall. The fall of Adam and Eve is why we have these diseases. This is part of the dysfunctionality of the human condition. It's like Jesus when he stood before Lazarus's tomb. He wept. Why did he cry? Because he was angry at death! Death exists because of the dysfunctionality caused by human sin. I get angry at times, but I can't allow myself to indulge in anger because it so easily turns into self-pity.

"I've learned that our help is not in our strength," Walter is talking so fast and with such enthusiasm that I have a hard time keeping up with my note taking.

"It's like Jeremiah says," Walter is a passionate preacher at this moment. He quotes Jeremiah 9:23–24: "'Let not the wise man boast of his wisdom or the strong man boast of his strength or the rich man boast of his riches, but let him who boasts boast about this: that he understands and knows me, that I am the LORD, who exercises kindness, justice and righteousness on earth, for in these I delight,' declares the LORD."

"Our hope is not in our own strength but in the restoration of all things, in the resurrection. Our bodies and the entire cosmos will be renewed. It is like that passage you cite from Revelation, Jeff, a text

I had previously overlooked, about the tree of life in the heavenly Jerusalem having leaves that are medicine for the healing of all these diseases" (Rev. 22:2–3).

"Paul talks about it in Second Corinthians," Walter says enthusiastically. "He talks about this earthly tent being destroyed. By 'earthly tent' he refers to his physical body. Paul is looking forward to the heavenly state, the resurrection state. He doesn't really look forward to the intermediate state of having no body, but he does look forward to the resurrection when we will have a new body free of disease, when the entire cosmos will be renewed! And that is what I look forward to.'"

A Unifying Theory of Spiritual Coping

There is an incredible diversity in how people use their spirituality to deal with illness. At first, it would appear that there is so much divergence in this chapter that there is nothing that these spiritual coping styles have in common. Can we find themes in this bewildering array of spiritualities? Is there anything that these people share as they cope with chronic conditions?

We can't say that sick people endure because God helps them, since some of the people in this chapter don't think of themselves as being in a relationship with God. Reverend Koshu would absolutely not use the name God when describing how he copes. Whereas Christians and Muslims see attachment to God as the path to salvation, Buddhists see detachment as the path.

Some readers, trying to understand this chapter, might arrive at the conclusion that all spiritual traditions are the same, since they all relate to the spiritual realm. That's fuzzy thinking. Only to a limited extent do I agree. Different forms of spiritual coping might have a positive effect on specific health risk factors, as I discuss below, but even though we can generalize about the health effects of spirituality, we cannot say that the major religions are similar in other respects. These religions teach drastically different things. Some spiritual traditions are mutually exclusive, so they can't all be compatible.

The pivotal question here is, How does spiritual coping impact health? I propose a unifying theory: Spiritual coping has a positive impact on a variety of health risk factors.[19] According to the theory I'm about to expound, risk factors are intermediate variables in the causal chain between spirituality and health. It is like a domino effect, and the middle dominoes are health risk factors. For example, altruism, a sense of well-being, tranquility, and optimism are all protective factors vis-à-vis health promotion and disease prevention.[20] Spiritual people are more likely than those who are not spiritual to be altruistic, to have a sense of well-being and tranquility, and to be optimistic.[21] Thus spirituality improves these protective factors, and these factors in turn improve the probability of health.

Spirituality also increases one's network of friends and community and increases the probability of following a doctor's orders and using seatbelts (because of a greater tendency to comply with authority). According to medical research, having a social network (strategy one), following your doctor's orders, and using seatbelts all lead to better health.[22] I am talking probabilities here, which is how we epidemiologists think.

There are risk-taking behaviors that could also be the middle dominoes between spirituality and health. Compared with those who are not spiritual, those who are spiritual are statistically less likely to smoke cigarettes or use alcohol to excess.[23] They are less likely to engage in dangerous health behaviors, such as using illegal drugs or engaging in promiscuous sex, and are therefore less likely to acquire sexually transmitted diseases.[24] They are less likely to get broken bones in barroom brawls, less prone to road rage, less apt to be violent, less likely to get divorced.[25] They are less socially isolated. Social isolation increases the probability of poor health (the converse of strategy one).

Of all the health risk factors, only one is influenced in the wrong direction by spirituality. Can you guess what? The answer, which may be obvious, is that spiritual people tend to be more obese than those who are not spiritual. This doesn't mean that all spiritual people are fat. Rather it means that, as a group, spiritual people are fatter. As one woman said when she read the previous sentence, "Well, what else are we allowed to do? If we're uptight and stressed, we're not allowed to get drunk or participate in an orgy or scream at someone. So we deal with our stress by stuffing our faces!" Another person said, "Why is it that church suppers serve such fattening food?"

This unifying theory—spiritual coping has a positive impact on a variety of health risk factors—fits the research data and also explains what the people you read about in this chapter share. The following table tests this theory against the four people whom I interviewed for this chapter. Health risk factors are on the left-hand side of the table; the four interviewees are across the top of the table.

Table 3

Testing the Unifying Theory

Health Risk Factor	Donna Joblonicky (life force)	Morris Days (Muslim)	Rev. James Koshu (Buddhist)	Walter Unger (Christian)
Has a chronic illness	yes	yes	yes	yes
Uses spiritual coping	yes	yes	yes	yes
Is altruistic	yes	yes	yes	yes
Has sense of well-being	yes	yes	yes	mostly
Is tranquil	yes	yes	yes	mostly
Has friends and community	yes	yes	yes	yes
Has coherent sense of meaning	yes	yes	yes	yes
Follows doctor's orders	yes	yes	yes	yes
Uses a seatbelt	yes	yes	yes	yes
Smokes cigarettes	no	no	no	no
Uses alcohol to excess	no	no	no	no
Uses illegal drugs	no	no	no	no
Is sexually promiscuous	no	no	no	no
Has barroom brawls	no	no	no	no
Is a violent person	no	no	no	no
Has fits of road rage	no	no	no	no
Is socially isolated	no	no	no	no

This table shows that our sample of four interviewees from drastically divergent spiritual traditions is almost identical in terms of spiritual coping and a wide variety of health risk factors. In the top half of the table the answer is yes to almost all the questions, and in the bottom half it is no to all the questions for all four interviewees. This table demonstrates a remarkable degree of convergence among the four people I interviewed for this chapter.

Thus the health effects of spirituality may not be so mysterious after all.

6

CHRISTIAN SPIRITUAL RESOURCES

The perspective of this chapter, which continues the exploration of spiritual methods of coping with illness, is exclusively Christian. This is because Christianity is not only the most popular spirituality, but it is also the one I ascribe to. Because of my identity as a Christian, most of the sick people referred to me for interviews are Christian. In this chapter I will focus on three strategies these interviewees taught me:

Strategy ten: Say the Jesus Prayer
Strategy eleven: Go to church
Strategy twelve: Change the world

Jesus says, "I am with you always, to the very end of the age" (Matt. 28:20). In this chapter we will focus on how a Christian's relationship with Jesus can provide the strength to pull him or her through tough times.

Strategy Ten: Say the Jesus Prayer

In the United States today, stress management experts in medical settings teach meditation, "mindfulness" (which is Buddhism), and a variety of relaxation techniques, but they overlook a stress-management technique that has been taught by the Christian church for the last one thousand five hundred years. Even Christian psychologists teach relaxation techniques rooted in the Asian religions and ignore the spiritual tradition I'm about to tell you about. It's called the Jesus Prayer. It consists of the following words said repeatedly: "Lord Jesus Christ, have mercy on me! Lord Jesus Christ, have mercy on me! Lord Jesus Christ, have mercy on me!"

Tom Powers Jr., who had severe heart trouble starting at age thirty, taught me about this prayer. Going by the nickname Dooley, he lives in Hankins, New York, on the banks of the Delaware River.

Faced with crushing chest pain and overwhelming anxiety, Dooley did not want antianxiety medications, because of a history of alcoholism. Yet he was between a rock and a hard place. If he allowed himself to think, he would be anxious, which could worsen the heart attack. Saying the Jesus Prayer allowed him to calm himself down without medications.

Here is how Dooley states the dilemma: "When you get into an acute situation, whether it is pain or a threatening level of illness or even emotional upset, when things just pile up, it is better to think less and pray more. In an acute situation you can't do much, and if you try to do anything, you are simply adding frustration to what is objectively unchangeable in the situation. The task is to endure pain and the unusual mental states that pain induces, without adding frustration and panic to the situation unnecessarily."

If the Jesus Prayer is repeated several hours a day, it has the capacity to block out pain, anxiety, and temptation. It lifts the human spirit out of the mire and into the heavens, without antianxiety or pain medication.

A lengthier version of the prayer is, "Lord Jesus Christ, Son of God, have mercy on me, a sinner!" Some monks in Russia and Greece have spent their entire careers studying this prayer, and they teach rhythmic breathing in connection with the prayer. Catholics have told me they derive similar stress management benefit from saying the Rosary.

The Way of a Pilgrim is a famous book, written in the 1850s by a homeless peasant in the Russian steppes.[1] We know very little about the author except that he is thirty-three years old and a widower with a crippled arm who is on a spiritual quest. He is in search of a way to pray continuously, as Paul prescribes in 1 Thessalonians 5:17. Our pilgrim explores various methods of interior prayer, finding that his mind wanders. Finally, he meets a spiritual director who shows him a classic text of Orthodox spirituality (the *Philokalia*) and there he discovers the Jesus Prayer. The spiritual director advises our pilgrim to repeat that prayer twelve thousand times a day. As can be imagined, for the first two days he finds this difficult. After that the prayer becomes habitual and it transforms his life, spiritualizing his everyday existence, filling him with cheer, and making him always conscious of God's presence.

This prayer is also known as the Prayer of the Heart. Professor Albert Rossi from St. Vladimir's Orthodox Theological Seminary says, "There is within us a space, a field of the heart, in which we find a Divine Reality, and from which we are called to live. The mind, then, is to descend into that inner sanctuary, by means of the Jesus Prayer or wordless contemplation, and stay there throughout our active day and evening. We descend with our mind into our heart, and *we live there*. The heart is Christ's palace. There, Christ the King comes to take His rest."[2]

Many Eastern Orthodox writers point out that the power of the Prayer of the Heart arises from its use of the name of Jesus, because there is power in that name (Matt. 12:21; John 14:13–14; 15:16; 16:23–26; Acts 2:21; 3:6, 16; 4:10, 30; 16:18; 21:13; Phil. 2:9–10; Heb. 1:4; James 5:14).

Tom Powers's Story

"At age thirty I had a heart attack," Tom says. "It later turned out that the diagnosis was wrong. It was not an infarct. I was in and out of the intensive care unit for a month. Finally a cardiac catheterization made it clear that it was a functional disorder. During that time I said the Jesus Prayer.

"My illness was a terrifying and life-changing experience. Up until then I had a teaching career and I was the assistant track coach. I had a wife and children. Then I developed chest pains. The doctor took one look at the EKG and then shot me up with enough Demerol to send me off to the planet Uranus. The doctors couldn't get my heart regulated. My pulse rate was down in the thirties, and my blood pressure was low.

"I told the doctor that I couldn't take mind-changing medications due to their addictive qualities," Tom continued. "I had been in Alcoholics Anonymous for six years at that point. I had a tendency to become obsessed and compulsive about booze and other junk, so I told him I didn't want mind-changing medicines. Only later did I discover that the doctor gave me sedating medicines contrary to my wishes. I was very nervous. I used the prayer method of trying to calm myself down. My AA sponsor taught me the Jesus Prayer, and I read the book *The Way of a Pilgrim*.

"Two weeks later, after I got out of the hospital, I had another attack when I was at home. I developed severe chest pain. My air supply was cut off. I hyperventilated. Everything went wrong at once. The oxygen tanks I had at home ran dry just at that minute, empty. An ambulance that was supposed to take me to the hospital got lost and couldn't find my house. I couldn't breathe. My dad thought I was dying. He kept telling me to pray. Because I couldn't breathe, all I could get out was the single word 'Jesus!' But that word of prayer alone put enough easement into the situation that I was able to hold out until the ambulance arrived.

"The doctors recommended surgery," Tom explained. "They expected me to die of heart disease within six to twenty-four months if I didn't have surgery. I was opposed. I have never liked the thought of surgery. Eventually I agreed to a cardiac catheterization. They wanted me to be conscious while they did the procedure so they could tell me to breathe when they wanted me to breathe. I couldn't imagine remaining conscious during such a procedure.

"The night before the cardiac catheterization I couldn't sleep. I kept getting up and down all night. I tried praying the way I had read in the book *The Way of a Pilgrim*. That got me through the night. So I did manage to go through the procedure while remaining conscious, as the doctors wanted. And it is God's mercy that I did it. The catheterization proved that the diagnosis was wrong. They discovered that I had a functional disorder and not degenerative coronary artery disease.

"After that I turned more to alternative medical sources," Tom continued. "But meanwhile my doctors had got me addicted to barbiturates, narcotics, and tranquilizers. There was a nurse named Maggy that I liked to talk to. I told her that I couldn't figure out what was wrong with me. I felt terrible and groggy, like when I used to be an alcoholic. I told her that I had forbidden the doctor to give me mind-changing medicines, so I couldn't figure out why I felt so groggy.

"Maggy informed me that the doctor had readdicted me to the very medicines I had forbidden him to give me. So then, to get rid of the addiction, I went cold turkey. I had to sweat it out for the next six weeks to get off those drugs. I was out of my mind with migrating pains and crashing depression. I couldn't think and had to borrow the brains of the people in my church to get through the medication withdrawal effects. I just kept saying the Jesus Prayer to get through.

"This prayer is my constant companion. I am not a person who is endowed with courage. This prayer bridges the gap and gets me through the tough times. I must have had eleven or twelve surgeries in the last six years, for things like fistulas. I don't enjoy going for surgery. The Jesus Prayer is what keeps me from having an unspeakable dread of the unknown when I'm about to go into surgery. I'm saying the Jesus Prayer as the anesthesia comes on and I go to sleep, and I'm saying it when I come out of anesthesia. It allows me to go through an ordeal that I am unable to escape. It makes my life manageable despite surgeries. I even find that I have greater conscious contact with God after one of these experiences.

"Periodically I have heart episodes. Just this last weekend my heart rhythm was off and I had to cancel everything because I felt so sick. You tried to interview me, Jeff, and we had to postpone the interview because my heart beat was so slow."

In Hankins, New York, along the banks of the Delaware River, there is a wonderful campus called East Ridge, which is the center for a program called All Addicts Anonymous (AAA). This is a spiritual program that successfully treats all forms of addictions, using a twelve-step model. Tom and his father, Tom Powers Sr., are the leaders. Tom is now sixty-four years old. His father is ninety-two and was a contemporary of Bill W. (the cofounder of Alcoholics Anonymous). When Tom Powers Sr. established AAA, he was influenced by the spiritual writings of the Russian Orthodox Church.[3]

"My AA sponsor is my dad," Tom explains. "He wrote a book called *Invitation to a Great Experiment*. The last chapter is about the Jesus

Prayer.[4] Mahatma Gandhi used this form of prayer. At an earlier stage of my life, Gandhi's life and work meant a lot to me. I've been a Christian all my life. Even when I was an alcoholic, I was still a believer. I value the wisdom of other religions, but it is the Christian religion that is all in all for me. The concentric prayer or centering prayer that has meant so much to me is the Jesus Prayer."

When I first met Tom, he and I had strolled across the lawn of the campus where he lives, among scattered cottages and a gigantic vegetable garden with the corn towering over us. Later, when I had scheduled an interview by phone, Gwen, his wife, had told me that Tom was unavailable because his heart was beating at thirty beats per minute, and he had gone to bed. The next time I scheduled a phone interview, he was available because his heart was better behaved.

"I once had cancer," Tom told me. "The doctors wrote me off again, saying I was close to death." Tom continues to talk about his cancer. "I had to go through medical regimens for twenty months, with continuous, intense pain. The pain was so bad that I couldn't read. I just stayed in my room for months with a damp cloth over my eyes, hanging on with the Jesus Prayer. I don't know anything else like it for producing joy in the midst of difficulty.

"There are three books about the Jesus Prayer that are important to me," Tom continues. "First there is my dad's book, *Invitation to a Great Experiment*. Then there is *The Way of a Pilgrim*, which is easy to read, like a Dostoyevsky novel. Then there is a book called the *Philokalia*. That book is some high-octane stuff. It is written by the Church Fathers. I read a copy translated by Kadloubovsky, called *Writings from the Philokalia on the Prayer of the Heart*.[5] It is difficult to understand. I almost have to be in a state of grace to crack the code.

"Christ didn't just say we should pray," Tom continues. "Christ said we should watch and pray. I take the word *watch* to refer to watching my mental sobriety and guarding my heart. This Jesus Prayer constitutes a whole-life study course."

Strategy Eleven: Go to Church

As I wrote in the introduction, medical research indicates that people who go to church or temple live longer and healthier lives.

Here is the story of a woman who is able to cope with chronic illness because of the help of her church and her pastor.

Charlene Slaver of Farmington, Maine, suffers from traumatic brain injury (TBI). When she was twenty-nine, her husband, Joe, was driving in a downpour. Their car hydroplaned at fifty-five miles an hour and crashed into a guardrail. Because of head trauma, Charlene developed severe memory deficits.

During the first year after the accident, Charlene was confused. She would get lost in her own house, unable to identify rooms. Sometimes she left pots cooking on the stove. She forgot how to tie her shoes, read, or spell her own name. Even as I write, three years after the accident, when Charlene signs her name, she occasionally forgets how to spell it.

Frustrated, Charlene took the laces out of her shoes. At least she could eliminate that problem! She began to leave notes reminding herself to do things, or she had Joe phone her to remind her. When she was cooking, she placed a piece of tape on the back of her hand, on which she wrote, "Stove On." That eliminated the fire hazard. Many people with TBI are taught to carry a notebook that serves as their memory. Charlene figured it out for herself.

Often that first year she would lose hours at a time, forgetting what had happened during them. Her daughter would say, "Mom, don't you remember that we did this, that, and the other thing in the last two hours?"

From Charlene's point of view, it wasn't that she forgot those things; she was sure they never happened. Other people's reality contradicted what Charlene knew to be true, because time for her just vanished. It made her feel like screaming and running away.

Charlene's church and pastor were instrumental in helping her through this trial. Often Rev. Earl Edgerly would meet with her and read Psalm 103 to her. Together they read it over and over. It became the Charlene Slaver Psalm. It begins: "Bless the LORD, O my soul: and all that is within me, bless his holy name. Bless the LORD, O my soul, and forget not all his benefits" (vv. 1–2 KJV). The psalm is so focused on God that it lifted Charlene's mind out of misery.

At times it seemed to Charlene that she had lost everything. She knew that she needed to cling to God, because in him she found stability and security. Friends from the church encouraged her, and her family stuck by her side. Amber Rose, Charlene's daughter who was eleven at the time of our interview, taught Charlene how to tie her shoes. At the time of our interview Charlene's shoes had shoelaces! Amber Rose also taught her to spell a few words. Her son, Joseph, and her husband, Joe, have surrounded her with tenderness.

Before the accident Charlene had begun to write an autobiography, but after the accident she couldn't remember most of it. Even though Charlene had publishers interested, when she read her autobiography, she could not remember all the abuse she had endured as a child. She could not remember having written it. The person described was no longer her. The story was foreign, as if someone else had written it. She began to understand that the Lord had delivered her from anger and torment by wiping those memories off the blackboard.

Almost sarcastically, Charlene had prayed that her life might become so busy that she would forget about herself, her troubles, and her pain. Through her church, this prayer was answered. Charlene began making what they called Boxes of Love for destitute families in the community. This was not motivated by pity but by faith. People on public assistance needed diapers, beds, and toys for Christmas. Church members began collecting such items and putting them in the boxes. One woman was going on a vacation to Peru. They found the name of a missionary in Peru and phoned to discover what that mission needed, so that the vacationer could take some needed items on the plane. Caught up in a whirlwind of church activities, Charlene was released from anguish and in the process was transformed.

"I forgot about me and stopped my whining, complaints, and fears," she says. "I focused instead on what the Lord wanted me to be doing at church. I began to pray and fast a lot. Even though my experience made no sense because of the gaps caused by amnesia, I trusted the Lord to make sense of things and provide direction. There are things I don't understand and need to accept, but I trust that God has a plan, and I find that his plan for me is better, more loving, and more fulfilling than I could ever have imagined. My life is his and is directed by him. God makes my life complete; I don't need to make it complete for myself."

With a determination not to be hampered by her memory deficits, Charlene began to work around them. That is the beauty I have discovered in writing this book. The heroes and heroines I interviewed have learned how to adapt to and work around the most unbelievable obstacles. It is a testimony to the strength of either the spirit with a small *s* or the capital *S* Spirit, depending on your point of view.

This illustrates something I will discuss in chapter 10, namely that TBI is different from the burden caused by TBI. The burden consists of the weight of the chronic condition crushing the human spirit. Whereas Charlene's TBI improved only slightly, her burden changed from heavy to light, because she learned how to prevent her condition from keeping her down. She learned to trust that if something was forgotten, it was not important. She was able to relax about the gaps in her memory, because whatever was missing was not necessary. If it was important to God, she believed God would cause her to remember it.

You might say that from Charlene's viewpoint she had two problems. One was holes in her memory, which we psychiatrists call a "swiss cheese memory." The other was anxiety about those holes. She could not accept having a brain that didn't work properly, so she was tormented. But when she began to accept herself as she was, her anxiety subsided. She learned to tolerate her imperfections.

People use various means to overcome their anxiety. Being a very religious woman, Charlene used the resources of the church to help her relax. Once the anxiety was gone, Charlene was able to function at full capacity, because one of her two disabilities was removed.

Many people with a permanent deficit aren't able to grasp this simple concept. "I would stop being so upset if my arm would stop hurting," one person tells me, failing to realize that being upset triples the pain in her arm. Another person says, "How can I stop being depressed if my leg doesn't work and will never work again?" As long as the focus is riveted on the leg, the person is paralyzed not by his leg but by his inability to view things from a different perspective. Such a person has three disabilities: depression, a bad leg, and a rigid way of thinking that prevents problem solving. That's part of what makes disease burdensome. Depression and rigid thinking are far more crippling than a bad leg. Often when we change to a positive perspective, despite our physical condition, our condition doesn't seem so bad.

During my telephone interview with Charlene, she talked extremely fast. My hand nearly fell off from fatigue taking notes. She said she was talking fast because she was afraid that she would forget something crucial. For days she had been praying that God would help her remember all the important things during the interview.

Charlene's memory has improved slightly over the last three years. For example, she no longer forgets things that happened five minutes ago. Her family has also helped her fill in the blank spots. Her sisters spent hours on the telephone with Charlene, reminiscing about the past. They also spent time with her poring over old photographs. Even though Charlene does not always remember, she enjoys hearing the stories. Slowly she has pasted together a collage of photos, memories, and other people's reports about her childhood, and now she thinks about her past with contentment and fondness, because the reconstruction of her childhood is more positive than the memories of abuse that she had prior to her accident.

"There are people worse off than me," Charlene says. "I have learned to stop saying, 'Why me?' Instead I now say, 'Why not me?' No matter what I have lost in my mind, I did not lose my church or my faith. God's awareness of me, his revelation for my life, is all I need. His grace, comfort, and compassion are true and steadfast. Praise the Lord!"

Like some others whom I interviewed, Charlene thinks of the accident as a blessing in disguise because it opened the way for a deeper relationship with God. Prior to the accident she was a Christian but lukewarm. Sometimes she was angry and depressed because of her childhood. Today she no longer remembers the anger and depression. Her church and her service to the Lord have become central to her life, and she believes this has more than compensated for her partial loss of memory.

Support

As I have interviewed sick people and unpaid caregivers, I've discovered that many of them find nourishment and encouragement in their church. Distilling that experience down to its essence, the most crucial reason that church is helpful is that in church we no longer feel alone. We have two kinds of allies: divine and human. It's difficult to determine where the human support ends and the divine support begins, because Jesus said, "Where two or three come together in my name, there am I with them" (Matt. 18:20). The support we experience is a combination of God's provision and the help of our Christian friends.

Epidemiological research finds a strong correlation between church attendance and health. As noted in the introduction, there have been more than thirty research studies demonstrating that those who attend church live longer and have more friends than those who don't.[6]

Research showing the health benefits of churchgoing can be criticized on the theory that people who get sick may no longer be able to get to church, so the association is not real, because those who become sickly drop out of church before they die. There are two ways of showing that this theory does not explain away the association between church and longevity. One way is by doing a prospective study in which you assess churchgoing at the beginning of the study, and then study mortality over subsequent years. In one well-designed, prospective study, the church-goers had a 41 percent lower risk of dying over the next seven years. In figure 8 you can see that those who do not attend church regularly die sooner than those who do. Seventy-eight percent of those who attend church regularly are still alive at the end of seven years, compared with 63 percent of those who don't attend church. Because this is a prospective study, the results cannot be explained away by saying that perhaps sick people stop going to church and that's why churchgoers live longer.[7]

Figure 8

Death Rate by Frequency of Church Attendance

(for 3,968 persons age 65 or older)

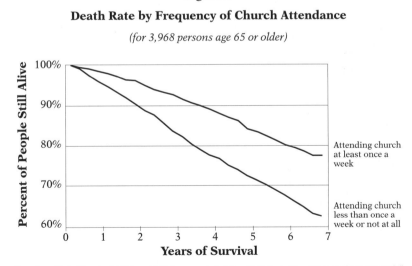

Data from H. G. Koenig, J. C. Hays, D. B. Larson, et al., "Does Religious Attendance Prolong Survival?" *Journal of Gerontology, Series A* 54A, no. 7 (July 1999): M373, fig. 1

A second way to demonstrate that there is a real relationship between church attendance and better health is the observation that when most people get sick or become disabled, they continue to go to church, finding transportation, if necessary, so they do not have to drop out. In a twelve-year prospective study, researchers at Yale Medical School found that "attendance at services is a strong predictor of better functioning," and "disability has minimal effects on subsequent [church] attendance."[8]

If you attend church, you are likely to have friends and acquaintances even if you have limited social skills. By "social skills" I mean the ability to remember people's names, say hello to strangers, start conversations, make small talk, show an interest in the other person, persist in holding up your end of the relationship, make phone calls, send emails, take the initiative, and so on. Not everyone has such skills. Shy people and those who feel rejected easily do better if they are members of a church where many people will be more tolerant of their idiosyncrasies. Research indicates that there is a difference in quality between the social network of churchgoers and those who don't go to church, so if you are timid, a nerd, or a social misfit, you will still have friends if you go to church. Even though Charlene can't remember the names of people at church, they remain her friends.

Strategy Twelve: Change the World

While many sick people find strength in church, they also find that spreading the gospel gives life meaning.

For her first eight years Arlene Pond was a running, jumping, tree-climbing child just like everyone else. When she was eight, she had three hemorrhagic strokes, which left her unable to use the left side of her body. She lost the ability to walk and talk.

Arlene doesn't remember those strokes. When she finally awakened after several brain surgeries, she had a tracheotomy and was on a respirator in an intensive care unit. The only part of her body she could move was her eyes.

Her immediate thought was, *What did I do that God is punishing me for?* She was convinced she must have done something to deserve such devastation. That's the way kids think. People explained that

God had a purpose for her life, but an eight-year-old is unable to understand such an abstract idea. Everything was terrifying.

Arlene's legs developed contractures. This meant that the muscles withered, and as they withered, they pulled her joints up into the position of frog's legs. After that her legs could not be straightened because of fibrous bands that grew inside the muscles. All four limbs were compressed into the fetal position. Her left leg and left arm were the worst, because the bleeding had been in the right side of her brain.

Arlene had several surgeries to straighten her legs, so that she would have some possibility of learning to walk again. Then the doctors put her in a plaster body cast that encased her entire right leg and half of her left leg and extended halfway up her chest. Her weight dropped from sixty-five to thirty pounds. Her left arm was considered to be beyond repair, and for the three decades since that time, Arlene has not been able to use it.

Arlene's brothers and sister came to the hospital a few weeks after she regained consciousness. When her youngest brother (age four at the time) saw her, he was frightened and did not know Arlene. He hid behind his mom and dad.

As she lay in bed for months in the total body cast, Arlene began to feel sorry for herself, wishing she were able to do the things she used to do, such as running and jumping or even walking. One day, when her father was sitting in the room with her, God spoke to her. That's how Arlene put it: "God spoke to me." She heard his voice say, "You are going to walk before your mother's birthday!" It startled Arlene. She looked at her dad but he was resting with his eyes closed.

"Did you hear that, Dad?" she asked, bursting into tears. Her dad said he had heard nothing. Arlene said, "God said that I would walk before Mom's birthday!" Her father looked bewildered and didn't say anything.

Arlene was convinced that God had spoken to her. Many readers may believe that God no longer speaks to people today as he did in the Bible. I have interviewed many people and found a half-dozen who say that they've heard God speak to them audibly, exactly as if someone were speaking in a human voice. With the voice, there comes an inner certainty: *This is God speaking.* While this is a spiritual experience, we must be cautious about declaring that all spiritual experiences come from God. There can be counterfeits.

When Arlene heard what she believed was God speaking to her, it was the turning point of her life. For her, hearing God's voice was a more decisive event than were her strokes and medical disasters. That experience shaped her life for the next three decades.

She heard: "You are going to walk before your mother's birthday!" and it was not just a future prophecy, it was a self-fulfilling prophecy. It motivated Arlene to work hard in physical therapy, to make the prophecy come true. That was no easy task. She had just four months, but with a walker, Arlene mustered her strength, grit, and determination and walked by her mother's birthday on August 29, 1970. Victory was exhilarating! By September she was able to return to school. That was incredible progress.

Arlene was in fourth grade when she rejoined her class. With the help of tutors who had come to her home, she had been able to keep up with her schoolwork. When she made her debut outside the hospital, she wore braces on her legs, her head was shaved, she was thin like a skeleton, and her left arm was withered. Also her voice (which she had recovered with speech therapy) sounded slightly ragged as if she had a touch of laryngitis. Arlene's classmates were astonished to see her.

At the time of our interview, Arlene was thirty-six. Her voice has retained that same ragged quality throughout the last three decades. Arlene has been through more than thirty surgeries. Her leg surgeries were focused on degenerative arthritis of her knees, because they had a lot of wear and tear from decades of being used in a way that was not as smooth as it should be. She has had many brain surgeries to relieve pressure inside a cyst that developed in the scar tissue.

Since age eighteen Arlene has lived independently in her own home. She works full-time as a medical secretary and has worked in almost all departments of the hospital. Currently she is secretary to the chairman of radiology at the Wright Patterson Medical Center on the Air Force base ten minutes from her house in Fairborn, Ohio. Arlene can type fifty-five words a minute using her right hand only.

She wears a brace on her left leg and is able to walk around her house with a cane. If Arlene falls, though, it is almost impossible for her to get up by herself. Her dad built her a lifting device, so that if she falls inside her house, she can scoot across the floor, get on the lift, and have an electric engine lift her to a standing position. She has phones in every room and a cellular phone in her pocket when she walks to the garage, so that she can always call for help if she has fallen in such a way as to be unable to get to the lift. From time to time she phones work in the morning, saying, "I've fallen, so I'll be late!"

"Do you want us to come help you?" they usually ask.

"No. I'm fine," Arlene invariably says.

Owning a home has been helpful. It allows her to adapt the house to her needs. The fifth strategy for coping with chronic conditions is: Avoid disaster. For Arlene it would be a disaster to lose her independence and become a burden to others.

For the past seven years Arlene has used a three-wheel motorized scooter for going long distances, such as when she walks her dog, Toby. The scooter fits easily into the hatchback of her Chevy Citation. Arlene drives her car with ease, using her right leg, which works fine.

She lives alone but is not lonely. To begin with, she says she experiences an immediate presence of the Lord, who is her comfort and companion. Her dog, Toby, is always fun, and wants to play ball with her as soon as she comes home from work. Like many people with a chronic illness or disability, Arlene has to spend much more time with the trivial details of life than do people without disabilities. For example, it takes her one or two hours to get ready for work in the morning. The amount of preparation varies depending on whether she can get her blouse on, whether her legs are in pain, whether she falls down, or whether all the parts and pieces of her body coordinate smoothly.

In the evenings she has started her own cottage industry of desktop publishing, making brochures and pamphlets for customers, such as the physicians at work. It brings in a little extra cash. Sundays she goes to church and is involved in a lot of church activities. It is a full and rewarding life. She wouldn't mind getting married, but there are no suitors.

You might think this woman has endured the tribulations of Job, but that isn't the way Arlene feels about it, nor is it the way she affects people around her. She is like a breath of fresh air for the people who work with her. She considers herself to be especially blessed by God and tells me that the good things God has given her far outweigh the disabilities.

She says that God is always with her and gives her life a sublime quality. Anytime she is in trouble or in a desperate fix, she says the Lord performs a miracle to rescue her. Arlene tells me that even her trials and tribulations are a blessing, for they give the Lord an opportunity to demonstrate—through miracles—how deeply he cares for her. Thus every adversity is like Valentine's Day, when she gets a love note from heaven.

The first "miracle" that Arlene became aware of occurred during her initial brain surgery, she tells me. She says she died on the operating table at age eight but was resuscitated. The neurosurgeons tied off the bleeding vessel twice, only to have it bleed again each time, causing more damage to Arlene's brain. When the artery was repaired a third time, the surgeons said, "We have done all we can. It's out of our hands." From that time on, Arlene has never suffered another cerebral hemorrhage. She believes that the surgeons put her arteries into God's hands, and that is why the vessel never bled again.

When Arlene heard God speak to her at age nine, she had a sense of being special. God doesn't speak to everyone! Arlene is amazed and honored that God would actually speak to her. This feeling of being special was reinforced when Arlene learned to talk and to walk, against all odds and contrary to what the experts had predicted.

Arlene is convinced that God (or a guardian angel) stands beside the surgeon every time she has surgery. For example, her orthopedic surgeon was about to make an incision when he abruptly changed his mind about where to cut. It turns out that he would have cut into a major blood vessel if he had followed his original plan. This proves that God was in the operating room, Arlene says.

She talks about a pact between her and God. When she needs special help or miraculous intervention, all she has to do is to ask for it. For example, once, when she was living in an apartment building, she fell down in the parking lot and was unable to get up. She was alone with no telephone. In an apartment near Arlene's lived a woman who worshiped the devil. The door to that woman's apartment was locked, but suddenly the wind blew the door open and the woman thought she heard someone knock on the door. She came outside to see who was there and discovered no one at the door but Arlene lying nearby in the parking lot. The woman helped Arlene to her feet, then said, "Boy, you sure have Somebody looking out for you!"

Another time Arlene fell beside the front step of her home and was stuck. She said, "Lord, you are going to have to send me some help!" Then Toby did something the dog had never done before and hasn't done since. He ran across the street, barking, running up and down the lawns of the neighbors, trying to get their attention.

"Whose dog is that?" one neighbor asked.

"It's Arlene's dog," another said. "We'd better go see if she's okay." So Arlene was rescued.

Because Arlene experiences the Lord as immediately present in her life, arranging things so they work out okay, she feels she is blessed. Whenever Arlene goes to surgery, as she often does, she is never sure that she will survive. But it really doesn't matter. Whether she lives or dies, she is in the Lord's hands, she says.

As is the case with most people who have a chronic illness, Arlene's future is unpredictable. Will she need a total knee replacement next year? Will she get a debilitating infection? All of us live with unpredictability about our future, but those of us who are healthy have an easier time denying the possibility of disaster, so we can live with the glib notion that our future is bright because that is what we have come to expect. Arlene is not able to be so carefree about the future and does not place her trust in her own health but in God. For Arlene the following verse is particularly meaningful: "No temptation has seized you except what is common to man. And God is faithful; he will not let you be tempted beyond what you can bear. But when you are tempted, he will also provide a way out so that you can stand up under it" (1 Cor. 10:13).

Every year she gets weaker and can do less than she used to. Her degenerative arthritis is causing pain in her knees. Her muscles are weaker than when she was young. Yet she is never alone, for the Lord is always present, providing for her needs. His presence more than compensates for her losses.

From time to time Arlene has an urge to phone a woman who suffers from chronic depression. Whenever she does, the woman says, "I'm so glad you called just now! I was feeling especially low today." That woman says that Arlene is more help than her psychotherapist.

Other people phone and ask Arlene to pray for them, because they believe she is especially close to the Lord.

"Why doesn't the Lord heal you of this affliction?" people ask.

"The Lord has healed me!" Arlene replies. "My primary purpose on this earth is to bear witness to the Lord's glory. For that purpose the Lord has given me an exterior frame that appears to be crippled and abnormal. The advantage is that people notice and stop to ask me how I can manage. Then I have the opportunity to hand them one of the pamphlets about my life, so that is an occasion to testify about what the Lord has done for me. If I didn't appear crippled, no one would ask, and I would not have the opportunity to testify!"

Arlene is using strategy twelve: Change the world. This strategy means that you use your illness as a platform to influence reality for other people. In the introduction I talked about my brother-in-law Chris Goffredo, who is using his illness as a platform for an environmental crusade against pollution. In the case of Arlene Pond, she uses her illness as a platform for spreading the gospel. This evangelization gives Arlene a sense of purpose and meaning. It is what keeps her going, the same way that Chris's environmental crusade gives him a sense of purpose and meaning, and keeps him optimistic.

She produced a two-page pamphlet that explains her history and tells many of the great things the Lord has done to show his special favor. She passes them out to anyone who asks about her condition. The chaplains at her hospital hand these out to motivate and inspire their patients who are discouraged with their plight. Her minister, Rev. Kenneth Milby, passes them out at church. This is the first step in fulfilling Arlene's calling, for she feels that the Lord has called her to bear witness widely.[9]

Two Bible passages that are especially meaningful to her are Romans 14:7–8: "For none of us lives to himself alone and none of us dies to himself alone. If we live, we live to the Lord; and if we die, we die to the Lord. So, whether we live or die, we belong to the Lord"; and Romans 8:28: "And we know that in all things God works for the good of those who love him, who have been called according to his purpose."

To all who know Arlene, she is a testimony of a positive attitude. When Dr. Townsend, a radiation oncologist, was in her office recently, he noticed the speed of Arlene's typing—fifty-five words a minute with 95 percent accuracy. He stood in the doorway and watched her using her right hand, her left arm thin, withered, and drawn up into a folded position. The physician stood there in the doorway and watched in amazement as this cheerful and delightful woman worked away with astounding efficiency.

Two years after I first interviewed Arlene, I phoned her to see how she was doing. In the interim Arlene had had two surgeries on the shunt in her brain, and a total right knee replacement. She continues to experience miracles. Her 1985 Chevy Citation died. She needed a new car that her scooter would fit into, but was thirty-eight dollars per month short of being able to afford the car payment. So she prayed for guidance. Arlene had forgotten that she was due a pay raise this year. The next paycheck was exactly thirty-eight dollars per month more than the previous paychecks. It was yet another Valentine card from heaven. She praised God. It's evident to all who know her that glorifying God, not sickness, is the defining feature of Arlene's life.

Winston Churchill, suffering chronic depression and alcoholism, led Britain to victory in World War II. Franklin Delano Roosevelt led America to victory despite paralysis from polio. Abraham Lincoln suffered depression. Seabiscuit's jockey, Red Pollard, had a severely injured leg when he rode Seabiscuit to victory. Julius Caesar, Napoleon, Alexander the Great, Charles Dickens, Peter Tchaikovsky, and Albert Einstein had epilepsy. Homer was blind. In each case, it was *not* the chronic illness for which we remember the person.

Similarly, Arlene wants us to remember her for her special relationship with God, for the double portion of the Spirit that the Lord has blessed her with, like Elisha. She does not want us to remember her for her medical disasters. What she wants is that we should listen to her, and through her, hear the gospel.

I was astonished by this woman's strength and courage. This morning when my alarm went off at 4 A.M., so that I would have time to write Arlene's story, I felt sluggish and sorry that I had to move my tired bones out of bed. But, if Arlene can get out of bed every day, so can I!

7

Grab the Bull by the Horns

This chapter will provide flesh and bones for strategies thirteen through sixteen:

Strategy thirteen: Take charge
Strategy fourteen: Take the medicine as prescribed
Strategy fifteen: Expect a cure
Strategy sixteen: Keep busy

The organizing principle of this chapter is that you should take an active role in dealing with your disease. Too often the word *patient* and the medical model reduce people to a passive role, like passengers on a roller coaster. Such passivity might be okay if you have a short-term medical problem, but over the long haul, you've got to be more in charge of your life.

Strategy Thirteen: Take Charge

Eileen Clarke of Middlebury, Connecticut, was asked to write a five-page paper about what her life would be like if she were something other than human. She wrote as an imaginary pancreas. She would talk to her friends, other pancreases, to figure out why some of them worked and others didn't. Her teacher gave her an *A* on the paper, then asked her how she ever arrived at such a fanciful idea.

Eileen's twin daughters, Kayla and Kelsey, who were almost eight years old when I interviewed her, have both had type I diabetes since they were fourteen months old. Neither girl has a pancreas that produces insulin. Why their pancreases stopped working is a mystery—there is no family history. There was a chicken pox epidemic at the time of onset, and this may be the answer. Medical researchers are investigating this virus as one of the culprits that may attack the islet cells of the pancreas and destroy them, causing diabetes. The flaw in the theory is that neither Kayla nor Kelsey had signs of chicken pox on their skin.

For several months after the chicken pox epidemic had subsided, both girls acted out of sorts, especially Kelsey. She became quite ill. A pediatrician kept shrugging it off as just "an average viral ear infection," or "just a normal diaper rash." But, call it a mother's intuition if you want, Eileen knew something was wrong, especially after Kelsey began projectile vomiting.

She took Kelsey to the emergency room of my hospital. The child was dehydrated. She had been drinking large amounts of fluid and urinating a lot, which was why she had the diaper rash. Kelsey had a blood sugar of over 900—sky high. When Eileen heard this, she burst into tears.

Kelsey was hospitalized for five days and started on insulin. On the day that Kelsey was discharged, Eileen did a fasting blood sugar test on Kayla. It was 183. Then Eileen knew that her intuition was right. She had two children with type I diabetes.

Most of the care for her daughters falls on Eileen, because her husband, Bill, works in New York City. With his commuting time, Bill is away from home fourteen hours a day.

Both Kayla and Kelsey are on insulin pumps. Every other day a new tube needs to be inserted into the girls' skin so the insulin can get in. Eileen or the girls test their blood sugar eight to ten times a day, to balance carbohydrates with the right amount of insulin, trying to maintain a precarious balance.

Eileen made a decision to keep a positive attitude about diabetes (strategy four), even though she is aware that diabetes could shorten the girls' lives.

"You never know what your lifespan is anyway," Eileen tells me. "You could step off a curb tomorrow and get hit by a car, so I don't choose to dwell on that. We simply focus on keeping life as normal as possible. Testing blood sugar and maintaining the right insulin-to-carb balance is simply part of the routine. We don't make the diabetes into a big issue. We don't let the girls get away with anything because of diabetes."

When one of Eileen's kids is acting nasty, she tests the blood sugar to see where the child stands. If her sugar is normal, then Eileen enforces the same rules as if the child weren't diabetic. She doesn't overindulge her children but raises them as normal kids.

I've met children who were overindulged by parents because the child had a sickness. Often such kids are nightmares—rude, demanding, and selfish. The parents of such a child say he or she needs to be given leeway because of the illness. I think such parents should follow Eileen's example. Even the Bible agrees with Eileen on this. Consider the following three proverbs:

- "A youngster's heart is filled with foolishness, but discipline will drive it away" (Prov. 22:15 NLT).
- "Don't fail to correct your children. They won't die if you spank them" (23:13 NLT).
- "To discipline and reprimand a child produces wisdom, but a mother is disgraced by an undisciplined child" (29:15 NLT).

Here is some more of Eileen's wisdom: "For me a big issue is getting the kids away from the TV. The shows on TV aren't appropriate. Occasionally Nickelodeon is okay, but I don't want them spending much time watching Nickelodeon. They have each other to play with, and they have full lives with dance, gymnastics, piano, Spanish, CCD, Girl Scouts, and ice-skating. So they don't need TV."

Eileen has pitched into the work of the American Diabetic Association (ADA) and the Juvenile Diabetes Research Foundation (JDRF). She has served on the board of the local branches of the ADA and won the prize for the East Coast as their top fundraiser. Every year she and her girls go to Washington to talk to members of Congress about finding a cure (strategy fifteen).

"Faith helps me get through the darker hours," says Eileen. "If no cure is found here on this earth, I know there will be a cure in heaven. I have a brother, Jimmy, who is in heaven after an accidental fire when he was eleven. When times get rugged, I sense Jimmy's presence, and that is comforting. And my grandmother. She was a quiet woman but reassuring. She passed on years ago. I feel her guidance."

The primary focus of Eileen's work is to maintain a positive, upbeat attitude and a team spirit around the girls. "They should not be treated as children who have a chronic disease. They are normal children who happen to test their blood sugar. They are still monsters at times. I try to keep the lines of communication open. At the beginning of every year I tell the teachers the difference in behavior that will alert them to low blood sugar in Kayla, which is different than how Kelsey will act with low blood sugar. I volunteer at the school as a room parent, so I keep up a dialogue with the teachers.

"My sweetheart is Vikki Mehan, the school nurse," Eileen continues. "Vikki and I are always on the same wavelength. The kids go to Vikki's office to have their blood sugar tested, and if it is a little high or a little low, she knows exactly what to do. She has a refrigerator with a snack for them, like maybe a mini–juice box with seventeen grams of carbs. Vikki is a godsend. When Kelsey first met Vikki, she kept saying 'You can't spell Vikki without spelling icky!' It was cute. My kids love her. Vikki even volunteered to babysit so that Bill and I can go out for an evening. It is a bit too much responsibility for other babysitters."

Eileen is a bundle of enthusiasm. She creates a team spirit wherever she goes. Not only does she know how to stir up support for fundraising to find a cure for diabetes, she also creates a team among the children's teachers, so that everyone is cooperating in the plan of making the diabetes a nonissue. As team leader, Eileen carries a cell phone and beeper. Even the two girls work together as team members. For example, one time when the family was about to stop at McDonald's for lunch, Eileen instructed both daughters to give themselves a bolus of insulin in preparation. Kayla had forgotten her insulin pump, leaving it home after changing her clothes. So she borrowed Kelsey's for the bolus of insulin before walking into McDonald's.

Eileen believes her children should be her top priority. "A lot of parents put everything in front of their children," Eileen says. "But

I believe that children have to come first. Otherwise they won't grow up to be able to reach their full potential as adults."

Many of the people I interviewed for this book, including Eileen, thought they should not be interviewed because either their problems were not severe, or they were not cheerful 100 percent of the time. Only after I listened to Eileen did I understand that for her family the diabetes is not a severe problem, but that is only because of Eileen's skill at managing it.

The Team Leader

Who is in charge of managing your disease? Is it your doctor or you? If your answer is your doctor, you are following the traditional medical model, which works well for short-term or life-threatening diseases but does not work for chronic diseases. An alternative to the medical model is the educational model. It was first used with diabetes. When someone takes insulin, he or she needs to test blood sugar several times a day and adjust the insulin dose accordingly. For this, the traditional medical model is not realistic. For example, if your family wants to go to McDonald's, it would not work to have to phone the doctor's office and wait four hours for a nurse to phone you back and tell you to give the children a bolus of insulin just before going into the restaurant.

When insulin was discovered, the educational model was discovered. It puts the patient in charge of managing his or her condition. According to this model, someone like Eileen is trained by health professionals to adjust the amount of carbohydrates and insulin, depending on the moment-to-moment blood sugar reading. Eileen is in charge of managing the disease. The doctors and nurses act as teachers and coaches, and hospitals employ someone called a Diabetes Teaching Nurse.

In the introduction you read about Walt Larimore's idea that your doctor is like the coach of a football team, but the team still needs a quarterback, which in this case is Eileen. In Larimore's book *Ten Essentials of Highly Healthy People*, he says, "You'll need a good primary care physician as your coach—someone who's a medical expert and willing to listen to you, to coach and advise you." But with a good doctor, you still need to be the quarterback of the healthcare team.[1]

The educational model does not mean that the expertise of doctors and nurses is ignored. Everything the medical professionals know about a disease can and should be imparted to the quarterback, and the coach should be available at a moment's notice. But realistically it is the sick person and caregiver who are present twenty-four/seven, whereas the health professionals are usually not on the scene. Just as the coach of the football team isn't on the field for decisions that need to be made in microseconds as to whether to throw a pass to receiver A or receiver B or to run with the ball, the healthcare professional is often not present for moment-to-moment decisions about healthcare. So a realistic management plan involves empowering the quarterback under medical supervision.

By the time you have lived with a chronic illness for a decade, you can usually tell us doctors things we don't know, such as,

- "I can't take such-and-such medication because I am allergic."
- "Different doctors debate whether the correct diagnosis is X, Y, or Z."
- "Taking medicines three times a day doesn't work for me because I always forget the midday dose."
- "Every time my relative visits I get so upset that my disease flares up."

There is another reason that sick people and caregivers might consider taking charge, namely that the medical system is flawed, at least in the United States. Many people get excellent care, some get poor care, and for many the care is uncoordinated or nonexistent. Forty-three million Americans have no health insurance at all. The U.S. Supreme Court endorses the rationing of health resources.[2] Our medical system is not designed to treat chronic illnesses.[3] It is designed to treat short-term "episodes of care." Only now are our computer systems in healthcare shifting from being focused on "episodes of care" to being focused on "patients."

In other words, the people who consume most of the healthcare resources—the chronically ill—are not the ones the system is designed to treat. For example, being forced to change doctors every two years because your health insurance changes is not a good way to manage a disease that persists over three decades. Yet this is what happens in America today when employers are constantly renegotiating health insurance contracts. There is no consistency in healthcare over time.

As I said before, the ways in which the American healthcare system needs to reform to meet the needs of patients with chronic illnesses is spelled out in the Institute of Medicine's influential book *Crossing the Quality Chasm*. That book is reshaping American medicine as of right now.

Consider someone who has several illnesses, takes half a dozen medicines, and has several doctors involved. You would hope that one of the doctors would act as team leader coordinating all this. But often, at least in America, this is not the case. Insurance policies, such as Medicare, often won't pay any doctor for the extra time needed to act as team leader. Each specialist you see is bombarded, working at top speed, seeing one patient every eight minutes. When you are in his or her office for eight minutes, you feel so pressured that you forget two-thirds of the questions you wanted to ask. In other words, the American healthcare scene is, for many people, chaos. No one coordinates care. You are left to beat your own way through the thicket with occasional oases of coherent care from this doctor or that therapist.

In the United States, if you have a chronic disease, you will probably have two choices. Either you become the person in charge, or you face incoherence in terms of healthcare coordination. Since we do not live in a socialist system, in which the state is going to take care of you, but in a capitalist system, you must take the initiative. If you don't take the initiative, unless you have an extraordinary primary care physician, you will be faced with a total lack of order in your healthcare.

The educational model is replacing the medical model as the preferred way of dealing with chronic illnesses. Therefore many people avoid the word *patient,* which implies passivity and powerlessness, and use the word *client,* which implies power, rights, and responsibilities.

I asked Eileen Clarke what would happen to Kayla and Kelsey if she were not in charge of their care.

"Things would get messed up pretty fast," she replied. "I've taught them things like how to measure their foods so they can get an accurate count of the carbs. We even measure the amount of milk they use in their cereal. As they get older, they will be able to take on more responsibility. Someone has to be in charge, either them or me.

"Kayla was admitted to the hospital recently because of viral meningitis. My husband and I stayed with her. She needed to have a parent to watch over her, because the nurses didn't know how to deal with an insulin pump. So I stayed twelve hours during the day and my husband stayed twelve hours at night. When Kayla said she just wanted me there, I stayed all day and all night. As a parent you put yourself on the back burner. We take care of our kids first."

If clients rather than doctors are the people in charge of chronic illnesses, then there is going to be a change in the culture of medical care. On average the perspective of clients (and of unpaid caregivers) differs from that of medical professionals. Clients usually respect doctors but are more interested than doctors in trying alternatives to medical treatments, such as herbs, spirituality, and Alternative Medicine.

Mary Ockenhouse and CAM

The case history of Mary Ockenhouse illustrates the shift to what I call a more herb-and-God-oriented treatment program, which often occurs when power shifts into the hands of the healthcare consumer. You might think that a person who turns to herbs and natural remedies must have only a minor illness, such as a cold virus, which can be treated with echinacea. But that's not always the case. Many people, such as Mary, prefer herbs and natural remedies, rather than chemotherapy and surgery, as a way to treat cancer.

Research by David Eisenberg and Ronald Kessler at Harvard University astonished the medical community. They found that conventional medicine is only one side of the picture of how Americans get their medical needs met. The other side is Complementary and Alternative Medicine (CAM), which is a vast and expanding part of the medical scene.[4]

For twelve years Mary Ockenhouse of Jim Thorpe, Pennsylvania, says she has managed to slow down or halt the spread of her lung cancer by means of herbs and a wholesome diet. She eats dandelion leaves, red clover, blue violet flowers, and an herbal laxative. In an effort to avoid chemicals, she has given up meat, coffee, and soda. She tried to give up tea but found she needed two cups a day of Lipton's, which she referred to as "my poison tea." She also allowed herself one soda a month.

When they first diagnosed lung cancer, the doctors said Mary had three months to live. That was fifty-six months ago. Mary figured, "If I have to die, I have to die." She refused chemotherapy or other medical treatments. Her fate was in God's hands, she figured. She reckoned that God put all kinds of pure foods and herbs on this earth for our benefit. Mary lives on top of a mountain, so she figured the dandelions and red clover were healthy because they were far removed from highways and not contaminated by chemicals.

It was the grape diet that seemed to make the biggest difference. For one month Mary ate only grapes and drank water. She allowed herself to eat as much of any kind of grapes as she wanted. Thus there was no hunger. A holistic doctor taught her to rinse the grapes in vinegar to wash off any chemicals sprayed on them and then to rinse them in water to get rid of the vinegar. After two weeks she was breathing better. She also increased her use of a Shaklee herbal laxative. Thirty days after starting the grape diet, she went back to her regular doctor, who took an X-ray of her lungs and found no evidence of tumor. She asked him about her grape diet.

"If it works, it works!" he replied. Unlike theologians, physicians are pragmatic.

Two years later the cancer metastasized to Mary's right eye, and then to her skull and brain. The doctors recommended surgery to remove her eye and part of her head. Mary declined, went home, and resumed her grape diet. This controlled but did not cure the cancer. The doctors predicted she would be blind within a matter of months. That was forty-eight months ago. She still sees fine out of both eyes.

"I went with the things that worked for me," Mary says. "You have to believe in what you are doing."

She has had two strokes in the last decade, but she is tough and determined to live in a way that makes sense to her. She refused surgery even though there was a tumor growing out the right side of her skull. It eroded the skull and compressed her brain. It was so large that she had to bend the right stem of her glasses so it curved around the tumor. She still has a large lump between her right eye and ear, with her glasses shaped to fit around it.

I asked Mary what keeps her so cheerful despite this twelve-year battle with cancer. She mentions three factors. First, the cancer has never caused much pain. Furthermore, although it caused an odd shape to her head, it didn't encroach on her lifestyle. As we talked, I could hear Mary sometimes breathing heavily into the phone, but that was due to her obesity not cancer. She grew obese because of her inability to walk or stand for more than a few minutes, because of an accident with a lawnmower four decades earlier.

Mary was accustomed to simply taking whatever life dished out, without complaint. I was reminded of another cancer patient who endured with stoic dignity years of pain from liver cancer. In his case the key was that he was a Marine. He said the Marines taught him to push his body to the absolute limit and beyond and then gather his determination and push further. That endurance served him well when it was his turn to live with persistent pain. He remained active and engaged with life as if nothing were bothering him.

Mary demonstrated her grit when her first husband abandoned her and her kids for another woman, leaving her with nothing, not even a car. She toughed it out, eventually marrying Richard Ocken-house, the man who drove her to church every week. Her patient endurance was again evident when she and her second husband decided to adopt kids from the Department of Children and Families. These kids came with extraordinary needs, having been abused or neglected. One infant was left by her mother in the parking lot of a grocery store. For more than a decade Mary and Richard never even left the house for a single cup of coffee together. In addition to her own three children, Mary adopted fifteen more. Many of them are now adults. Mary can see what a difference love and discipline have made in their lives.

Mary's faith has also helped her to be cheerful through the cancer ordeal. She was raised Baptist but joined the Church of Christ. That's how she met her second husband, Richard, who was converted in Germany and now preaches at her church. Hesitantly Mary spoke about how God was the key to her victory with cancer. Her experience was that most doctors had no interest in spiritual things, so she didn't know if she could trust me. Like many Christians, she feared being ridiculed. That's the reason most medical professionals never heard how central God is in her life.

"I don't talk about God because they might figure I was a wacko," Mary says.

I asked Mary which was more important, herbs or God. Immediately I realized that it was a dumb question. Mary draws no distinction between herbs and God. Herbs come from God. Eating a sensible diet and living by faith alone are two sides of the same coin, according to her way of thinking.

"God put these things here for us," she said. "Did you know that the needles from a pine tree are loaded with vitamin C?"

At the time I didn't ask Mary if she ate pine needles. I couldn't imagine eating pine needles. They would irritate my throat. A grape diet sounded plausible, but my body would rebel against a pine needle diet. Two years later, still obsessing about the pine needle diet, I phoned Mary and discovered that she'd never eaten pine needles. She laughed and said it was simply something she'd heard.

When I interviewed Mary, I thought she was so committed to herbs and natural treatments that she would refuse all traditional medicines. I was surprised to learn that she takes four drugs daily: verapamil, Plavix, Synthroid, and glyburide. She supplements the Synthroid with an herb that helps her thyroid. She also takes herbal antibiotics, and vitamin E. This is typical of Americans. The choice between conventional and alternative medicine is not an either-or decision. It is a both-and decision, as you can see when you walk into a pharmacy and see prescription drugs and herbal remedies side by side. It is actually more accurate to use the term *Complementary and Alternative Medicine* than just *Alternative Medicine*, because natural herbs are often used to complement conventional medicine. Many doctors don't know the extent to which their clients use unconventional approaches, because the clients don't tell the doctor about that sort of thing. Research indicates that CAM is a vast and growing aspect of the healthcare scene, as I mentioned above. I figure this is because of the increasing demand for all sorts of treatments (conventional and alternative), which is driven by the growing epidemic of chronic illness. The doctors' offices are flooded with patients, and so are the CAM offices.[5]

Mary concluded our conversation by saying that she has such bad scoliosis that two neurologists told her that her spine would shortly "snap in two," leaving her paralyzed from the neck down and on a respirator. "I don't worry about it," she said. "I don't know when it will happen, but there's nothing I can do about it anyway. I'm just grateful for the blessings I have, like a good husband. Richard and I make a great team!

"I'm so glad, Dr. Boyd, that someone is bringing God back into medicine," Mary added. "He was considered dead for a long time. I can't wait to read your book."

Like Eileen Clarke, Mary Ockenhouse is her own healthcare quarterback, taking charge of her chronic illness and medical care, and is taking a proactive stance, refusing to be passive.

Strategy Fourteen: Take the Medicine as Prescribed

Research indicates that patients swallow less than half the pills that are prescribed by doctors. This is true of the medicines for any chronic condition, from antidepressants to cancer medicine to blood pressure pills and blood thinners. Usually people take the medicine for a week after seeing the doctor, and then again for a few days before their next visit to the doctor. The majority of people who take their medication irregularly do not have lives that are as rewarding as the man I'm about to tell you about, who actually takes the medicine as prescribed.

Richard Geiger is a software engineer in Silicon Valley, California. He is also a Buddhist. Depression has played a significant role in Richard's life, causing him to be hospitalized twice and on medication. Fortunately, he has never attempted suicide. His wife and daughter have also had bouts of depression.

Richard describes what it's like when he is profoundly depressed: "I get very despondent and hopeless. Everything is awful and will always be awful. Nothing is enjoyable. There is a pervading blackness. My sleep patterns are disrupted. I lose my appetite, but I don't lose weight because I get physically inactive, so I burn fewer calories."

Richard has another chronic illness. Something is wrong with the long nerves that go from his feet to his spine. There is static in the wires. Richard experiences many unusual sensations in his feet, ranging from odd feelings to electrical jolts to pain. The antidepressant medicine he takes, along with Neurontin (gabapentin), soothes these nerves, reducing the extent to which he is jangled by bizarre sensations in his feet. The cause of this nerve problem, like the cause of depression, is unknown.

When Richard is depressed, it is helpful if his wife, Janet, just wants to be with him, not trying to convince him things aren't as bad as they seem. The experience of being loved, of having someone who is willing to sit with him, is comforting. That allows him to mobilize his own resources, so that he begins to think his way out of the maze of depression.

Richard says the depression is not just in the mind but also in his body. Therefore help can come from either direction. Richard finds that medicine makes a huge difference in his ability to sustain a positive outlook on life. Currently he takes Effexor (venlafaxine). I'll talk more about it later. This medicine, like Buddhist philosophy, allows Richard to feel that things are going to turn out okay. On the physical side, Richard finds that exercise helps to lift his spirits.

When he is despondent, Richard says that even the smallest details of life can confirm the apparent validity of his depression. If he gets in his car to go to work and finds that he has forgotten the car keys, it feels like a confirmation that life is miserable, that everything is conspiring against him. Then the Buddha's teaching about *duhkha* (suffering) pops into his mind and he has to laugh. The absence of car keys proves the First Noble Truth of Buddhism, namely that things are not the way he wants them to be. The specific causes and conditions of things lead to frustration, such as having no car keys. The purpose of the First Noble Truth is to help Richard realize that his happiness does not hinge on car keys, that he has choices about how he experiences life. The fact that he has these choices is central to Richard's thinking.

"Buddhist meditation allows me to sit and examine my thoughts," Richard says, "so that I understand how my mind operates, and I can recognize that these thoughts are not me. I can choose to embrace certain thoughts or allow other thoughts to pass by without bothering me. In the process I have become aware of the small twists and turns of thought that lead in a negative direction and are the first step down the road to depression."

Richard teaches his eleven-year-old daughter Lani to do the same thing. For example, a friend gives Lani a gift of thirty packages of trading cards. Richard wants Lani to have only a few packages today, so as to extend the excitement and pleasure over many days. But Lani wants all thirty packages immediately. She gets agitated. Instead of enjoying the trading cards, Lani comes close to feeling miserable.

"She is asleep to the idea that she could be happy at this time," Richard says. He suggests that she remember that she was happy this morning, and that it is up to her whether she chooses to embrace her frustration or the happy feelings from this morning.

Loving and respecting her dad, Lani takes his suggestion to heart and remembers that she has choices about how she experiences the trading cards. Her dad is right that she was happy a short while ago. If she feels agitated and upset now, she can decide whether or not to go with the frustrated feelings. She does not need to identify with those feelings.

This shows how Buddhist mindfulness can work and how it helps Lani avoid walking down the path of depression. It is like the Serenity Prayer: "Grant me the serenity to accept the things I cannot change, courage to change the things I can, and wisdom to know the difference."

A Pill for Depression

I am a psychiatrist, and I've found many patients are helped by antidepressant medicine the way Richard is, but many hate taking pills. As soon as they feel better, they stop the medicine. Then they get depressed again. It occurs to me that Richard is a thoughtful guy, attentive to subtle twists and turns in his private thoughts and feelings. I wonder what he would tell my patients about taking a medicine for depression.

When I ask him about it, Richard replies, "Off the medicine, I can tell the difference. If I forget to take it for a couple of days, there is a physical sensation inside me that is missing. In our meditation we Buddhists are trained to attend to sensations in the body. On the Effexor there is a very subtle but quite pleasant sensation, associated with that sense of the 'okayness' of things. It is the ability to set all worries aside for just a moment and feel happy in the present, without any reference to past or future. Off the Effexor that pleasant sensation is absent. I wish antidepressant medicine would work that well for everybody. The medicine allows me to relax and let go. The day goes better when I take these pills. Compared to the side effects that came with the older antidepressants," he continues, "this one is much better. I used to take Ludiomil, but I'm not sure if it's still on the market. Antidepressant medicines have come a long way. There are many less side effects than there used to be."

"How do you feel about having to take a pill to feel okay?" I ask.

"My only qualm about feeling dependent on the medicine is that I sometimes worry how I would do if I had no access to these pills. I've simply decided not to worry about that now. If in the future I'm unable to obtain this medicine, I'll deal with it at that time. I know I would then face a completely different situation. I would have an opportunity to discover whether more hours of meditation could have the same effect as Effexor."

"Some people tell me they feel humiliated at having to take antidepressant medicine," I say. "As soon as they feel better, they stop it, but after a while they get depressed again. What would you say to them?"

"I suppose I would ask them if a diabetic would feel humiliated taking insulin," Richard replies. "There is nothing humiliating about it. It is simply a choice I'm making, one of the many choices I make every day to take my life in a more positive direction."

Research indicates that only one depressed person in five gets treated for his or her depression; nevertheless effective treatments are available.

A week after our interview, I receive an email from Richard. It reads:

```
I did have a thought about another way to help somebody
to see how taking a mood medication is nothing to feel
humiliated over.

I suffer from another debilitating disease I forgot to
mention to you. It is a disease that would have been
crippling in past millennia. If there were not such an
effective treatment for this disease at present, I would
likely be considered disabled. I suffer from myopia.

I remember the day, at about age ten, when I received my
first pair of eyeglasses. I was shocked with delight! The
world was infinitely richer and more full of detail than
I'd known or suspected!
```

The glasses correct a defect of perception, caused by an
inherited condition. They allow me to perceive the world
with a visual clarity. My very livelihood depends on it.
They also allow me to take in beauty that, at times,
seems perfectly sufficient as a "reason to live."

Perhaps it's a commonly used analogy, to compare an
antidepressant or other mood medication to corrective
lenses. It does seem apt. In my experience, antidepressants certainly don't end suffering, any more than
clear vision eliminates seeing ugly or unpleasant sights.
But, just as glasses allow me to see unpleasant sights
more clearly, the medicine helps me to "feel" the world
more clearly than I otherwise would. And it turns out, I
believe, that my depression happens, in large part, due
to "emotional misperceptions": often "feeling" things to
be much worse than they actually are, which leads me to
behave in ways that tend to reamplify the misperception.

We constantly interpret the world. In Buddhism, "thinking" is considered a sixth sense faculty, after the
traditional five. Considered this way, one's thinking,
that is, the thoughts one chooses to recognize as the
"true picture" of the world, can be distorted, the same
way myopia distorts my sense of sight. Meditation helps
us to understand, at a very deep level—sub-verbal, at
least—that one's thoughts are merely spontaneously arising
propositions, to be tested, and accepted or rejected,
rather than somehow being an extension of a bounded self,
irrefutable.[6]

I am left with the impression that Richard is a thoughtful man who
has mobilized many resources to deal with his recurrent depressions,
such as exercise, meditation, and antidepressant medicine. He is a
software engineer to the core, which is fitting for a man who thrives
in Silicon Valley. Not only is Richard interested in how to rewrite
the operating system so as to allow the computer to function more
efficiently, he is also interested in how Buddhist "mindfulness" allows him to rewrite the operating system of the brain so as to allow
a person to function more efficiently. Richard is able to reprogram
his or Lani's mind in such a way that the glitches are eliminated and
harmony is restored. But, unlike a computer, the human mind can be
affected by a third element in addition to the software and hardware.
The third element is antidepressant medicine.

Reasons for Not Taking Medication

I am using Richard as an illustration of the idea that life is better if someone with a chronic illness actually takes the prescribed medicine. This strategy differs from the other nineteen. The other strategies in this book focus primarily on improving your feeling of well-being even though you continue to be afflicted by the illness. This strategy offers the possibility of changing the course of the illness itself. I have observed that the majority of flare-ups and relapses of chronic conditions are due to stopping the medicine, which most people do at least half the time. Sometimes this is because of side effects or the expense of the medication—things the patients failed to discuss with their doctor. More often it is simply because of neglect, as if they couldn't put a priority on taming the beast.

When a depressed woman comes to me for treatment, she might complain of trouble sleeping, no interest in sex, low energy, feelings of worthlessness, and suicidal thoughts. Being pessimistic, she is pessimistic about medicine also. Indecisiveness is part of the depressive picture, because she is thinking, "Life is bad, but if I take this medicine, it could be worse." Eventually, after careful negotiation, I get her to take the medicine. Next time I see her, I find she stopped the medicine because of side effects.

I ask her, "What side effects?"

She replies, "Trouble sleeping, no interest in sex, low energy, feelings of worthlessness, and suicidal thoughts."

I point out that she had those problems before starting the medicine.

There are many reasons for noncompliance with a doctor's prescription. Some of my patients have paranoia that is controlled by medicine. But one day the pharmacy switches the generic brand that it carries, and the white pill the patient was accustomed to turns into a yellow pill. The patient is not sure but suspects that maybe someone is trying to poison him, because the pill should be white not yellow. He's no fool! What do they take him for, an idiot? It's insulting that "they" think they can substitute a yellow pill without his noticing. So, quietly, so as not to attract the attention of the CIA or FBI, the patient stops taking the yellow pill. Pretty soon he is convinced that the yellow pill clearly is poison, and that means the other pills might contain cyanide also, so he stops all of them.

About a month later he notices an odd taste to his food, and decides it is safer not to eat than to die of poison in his food because of the conspiracy between the FBI and Mafia to murder him. A week later he is admitted to the hospital. He's dehydrated because he stopped drinking water when it tasted strange. The emergency department doctors give him intravenous fluids. Then he's admitted to my service (behavioral health).

Talking to this patient is not going to change his mind. He's certain his life is in danger. He avoids the hospital windows because a sniper might assassinate him with a high-powered rifle from a mile away. It takes us days to convince him to eat, and the only food he will accept is food that comes in closed containers so he can be sure the Mafia didn't tamper with it. A week later he decides to try taking medicine but only if it comes in a closed container so it is "safe." Eventually, after taking the medicine, the patient does 100 percent better. He enjoys going to the window to soak up some sunshine. Soon we discharge him back home. He has no overt paranoia. Life is delightful for him again. He lives in a safe world. But then six months later, to save money, the community pharmacy switches the generic manufacturer, and the yellow pill turns into a blue pill.

One man I treated did so well on his medicines that he decided his chronic illness had gone away. For months he continued to do well, which confirmed his impression that he was cured and no longer needed to take medicine for his bipolar disorder. Not only was life good, he felt increasingly happy, euphoric. On a mood scale from one to ten, he was a fourteen. He was more creative and sexier, felt abundant self-esteem, had boundless energy, and needed less sleep.

Mania, the disease from which he suffered, is characterized not only by euphoria but also by poor judgment. One day the man had a brilliant idea that was so hilarious that he simply had to do it. He decided that he should fly around the world. With an American Express card in his pocket, the trip was possible. Getting on an airplane in Los Angeles, he flew to Thailand. Changing planes, he flew to India. Changing planes, he flew to the Middle East. Changing planes, he flew to Europe, then New York, and back home. He landed in Los Angeles thirty hours after he departed. But he was so euphoric, agitated, and talking so crazy that the police took him to an emergency room where he was admitted to a hospital and treated with medicine that subdued his mania. Within a few days he returned to his right frame of mind but still laughed when he thought about his trip. Normal life would then have resumed, but when the credit card bill came in, his wife left him.

Here's another reason that people stop taking effective medicine. With the skyrocketing cost of drugs these days, medicines are becoming a bigger line item in the household budget than car payments or college tuition. Some families feel they must decide which half of the medicines they will buy, because they can't afford them all. If you are unable to buy all of your prescriptions, you should enlist the help of your doctor in prioritizing the list.

It is not just people with depression, paranoia, or bipolar disorder who are stubborn about medicines that have proven to help them. How many people do you know who have had a stroke or heart attack because they neglected to take their blood pressure and cholesterol medicine most of the time? How many recurrences of breast cancer are caused by failure to take the tamoxifen? Depression, paranoia, and bipolar disorder are only three of many diseases that would be much better controlled if people would simply take their pills as prescribed.

Physicians complain among themselves that patients are compulsive about taking their herbs and megavitamins three times a day, even though there is usually no evidence that these help, whereas the same patients can't be bothered taking their prescription pills as prescribed, even though those medicines have been proved to be effective. If you need a reminder to take your medicine, set the alarm on your watch or ask someone to phone you at work to jog your memory, or get a pill box with compartments for A.M. and P.M. pills for each day of the week.

Strategy Fifteen: Expect a Cure

Diseases that today are incurable may be cured tomorrow. You will be happier if you look forward to that tomorrow, even if it occurs in heaven rather than on earth.

When my barber, Placido Mastroianni, heard I was writing this book, he said, "That's me, Doc! Being sick well, that's me. Why not interview me?" So while he washed and clipped my hair, his story unfolded. Placido had a small stroke twelve years ago, affecting his right hand with which he cuts hair. One day when I went for my haircut, he had another barber there cutting hair under his supervision. Before, it had been a one-man shop. Over the next year Placido almost entirely recovered from his stroke. The only remaining deficit was that his boccie score was lower. Losing his competitive edge in boccie was a terrible blow to Placido. If he had been given a choice between permanently losing his ability to cut hair and having a lower boccie score, he probably would have retired as a barber.

He was diagnosed with coronary artery disease and had two stents. He also had a blockage in the artery to his intestines, an artificial graft to that artery, and now has radioactive pellets in his prostate because of cancer, and a gastric ulcer. His primary problem, as I see it, is hardening of the arteries.

"The reason I remain happy," Placido said, "is because I want to make the most of the years I have ahead." Placido is sixty-eight.

"Also," he continued, "I am hopeful because I expect they may discover a cure. Medical science keeps getting more advanced. I know people who have had problems, and the doctors were able to make the problems go away."

Placido has a magnetic personality. Over the three decades that he has cut my hair, he has always remained exuberant and loves to talk. More than half of each session is spent with him looking in the mirror so as to make eye contact with me and gesturing in the air with his scissors in one hand and comb in the other. I've always been afraid he might stab me when he gets animated in conversation, which is often. But he never has.

Pondering what Placido told me, I asked him about medication. He is on Medicare, which at that time provided no coverage for the six or eight different kinds of pills he took every day. "I'm living on samples, Doc," he said.

When my first wife was still healthy, before I went to medical school, Placido was my barber. He has been there through the decades. He was my barber when my son Justin died. During the years when I was at the National Institutes of Health, I would sometimes drive from Washington to New Haven to have Placido cut my hair. He does a good job.

Over the last three decades I've learned that Placido's wife has Huntington's chorea. At least one of his three children carries the gene. He told me his wife is getting irrational, berating him when he sets limits on what she can do.

"Placido," I asked, "if you are hopeful about a medical cure for your health problems, what about your wife's Huntington's? How do you remain upbeat about her?"

"Oh, there's nothing to be done about that," he replied. "When she gets irrational, it doesn't bother me much, because I know that it is an illness. Really my life is pretty good. I have these problems, but I feel okay and I'm still able to cut hair at age sixty-eight. So I have no complaints."

Expecting that a cure for your illness will be discovered is a lot more tolerable than accepting it as incurable. That is why the American Cancer Society sponsors so many fundraising events for "survivors." The American X Association, where X is the name of a disease, is usually seeking to raise money and public awareness in favor of "a cure for X." They follow the latest research, go to Washington, and lobby Congress in favor of finding a cure.

Dr. Steve Aronin, a physician in my hospital, treats people with AIDS. When he informs someone that he or she has AIDS, Steve does so in such a way as to foster hope. Hope is tender and fragile and needs to be cultivated. It is one of God's blessings, one of the three spiritual virtues discussed toward the end of chapter 5. It should be cherished and protected from harm. In the larger scheme of things, hope is realistic no matter how bleak the present appears to be. I will return to this theme at the end of this book.

I asked Placido how he would do if he were told that his illnesses were incurable.

"I would be discouraged," he replied. "Because hope is what keeps me going. That's why I fight to get better, because I have hope of a cure."

Philip Holladay's Cure

I met Philip Holladay of Beaver Falls, Pennsylvania, at the annual meeting of the Evangelical Theological Society. When he heard I was

writing this book, he was interested. Many people with chronic illnesses get excited when I tell them about my idea for this book.

Philip told me about his illness. The more I heard, the more flab-
bergasted I was. In the end, his story left me speechless.

Throughout his childhood everyone expected that Philip would die
of asthma, so no one got emotionally close to him. He was isolated
and left alone to struggle daily with the possibility of death. Against
all odds Philip survived. Eventually new medicines were discovered
that all but cured his asthma so that at age forty-seven he began to
lead a normal life. He was never troubled by the thought, *Why me?*
Since his asthma began at age two, he always accepted wheezing and
coughing as the way life was. For him, that was normal.

There was no family history of asthma, but as far back as Philip
can remember, he had to fight to breathe. Once he was sitting in
a doctor's office while his mother was temporarily elsewhere. The
nurses and doctors got alarmed about his breathing and began intensive treatment to keep him from dying. When Philip's mother
returned, she laughed. "That's the way he is every day; that's normal," she said.

Philip knew he was a mess. That was just the way it was.

Most of the time his parents were stoic. Although they did all the
correct things to take care of his physical needs, they never talked
with Philip about his asthma. They kept him at arm's length, neglect-
ing him emotionally. Once in a while his mother would look at him,
burst into tears, and run from the room, sobbing. No one ever talked
about why she did it.

All by himself Philip had to compete with death. He was always
coughing up large amounts of mucus and gasping so loudly that
everyone in the house could hear him. Death, which seemed to be
stronger than this little boy, was toying with him, like a cat teasing
a captive mouse. During the day Philip used an inhaler every five
minutes to be able to breathe for another five minutes. There was
an endless cycle of short-term relief from inhalers.

Every bedtime Philip would take pride that he had survived the day.
Night was another wrestling match with suffocation. Every twenty
minutes he would wake up with severe coughing to clear his lungs
of mucus. Every morning he was astonished that he had survived
the night.

Two younger brothers were born, two-and-a-half and three-and-a-half years his junior. They were healthy. One day, when Philip was old enough to understand, he made a conscious decision not to play with them, lest the world reject them as it had rejected him. Looking out the window, he watched them play together on the grass. He yearned to join them, but he was disciplined and stayed alone in his bedroom, crying.

People would stare at this boy who made so much noise coughing and wheezing. But no one made eye contact with him. There were two kinds of people. Kids laughed at, teased, and tormented him. Adults said, "Oh, gross!" or "Poor kid!" and backed away. He had no friends. At school he excelled at mathematics, something he could master without interacting much with humans.

In his childhood Philip's worldview could be summarized in six words: There is no love in humans!

When he was fourteen, in junior high and walking from one classroom to another, he suddenly stopped breathing. He was simply unable to gasp any more air. Alarmed, he rushed out onto the grass, took hold of a flagpole for support, grew weak and numb, and his vision dimmed. Within minutes he would be dead. A thousand kids walked past this dying boy. Everyone looked, but they all turned away from his gaze. As Philip was suffocating, he gave up on the human race. He wanted nothing to do with these people who did not bother to call the school nurse whose office was just fifteen feet away. Philip had always gone to church but didn't take it seriously. He didn't know if there was an afterlife. He hoped there wasn't. If there were an afterlife, he wanted to be alone, with no humans to annoy him. Then suddenly, against all odds, air poured into his lungs. Philip survived. Perhaps his bronchial muscles simply relaxed.

After that experience he gave up entirely on humans. Not telling anyone about his near-death experience, he avoided all conversation, even with his family, except for the occasional word or two that was unavoidable. He shunned all people. Having always been alone, he found isolation comfortable.

At age seventeen Philip decided that people had invented the idea of God to comfort themselves. He was sure of it. But there was a fly in the ointment. Being a mathematician, his logical mind objected that he had just made a statement without any empirical evidence to support it. So he decided that, while he couldn't disprove God's existence, he would find flaws in the Bible. So he read Scripture from Genesis to Revelation. But his plan backfired.

Philip lived in a loveless world. In the Bible he discovered love. He realized it was something he wanted to be part of, to be capable of loving people. (At this point it never crossed his mind that anyone could ever love him.) One night in bed, Philip prayed and said that he wanted to belong to Jesus Christ. And so he was born again. Had the gospel been brought to him by a living person, Philip would have rejected it. Only in book form could it penetrate through his aversion to humans and lodge in his heart. After his decision to receive Christ, he joined a Bible study with some guys who in the past had attempted to strike up conversations with him. He was amazed when he realized that someone from the Bible study sat beside him in virtually every class.

He decided he had to learn how to relate to people if he was going to love them. At a minimum, he needed to be capable of exchanging a few words. *How do you carry on a conversation?* he asked himself. This was unknown territory. He observed how people talked to one another. He learned a few stock questions, like "What classes are you taking this year? Who do you have for a teacher? Where do you live?" Armed with these questions, he was able to conduct brief conversations. A triumph! Mostly he listened—and learned about human discourse.

When he went to church, Philip found it meaningful and inspiring, and before long he emerged as a leader. While he majored in mathematics at North Carolina State University, he served as a youth pastor. He earned a Ph.D. in applied mathematics at the same college. Church provided a wide range of activities in which Philip exercised his leadership skills. Although he became active socially, he made a conscious decision not to date any women. His self-concept remained the same: *I'm a mess!* Therefore he never thought of marrying, so logically he couldn't date. And he didn't.

When Philip was twenty-six years old, Vanceril (beclomethasone) became available as a research drug—not available to the public. It was prescribed for Philip, and for the first time in his life, his asthma became less severe. He continued to wheeze and cough but less so. The drug changed his life, and he realized he might survive for a while. It was the first time he had allowed himself to look forward to a future. Although he still said, "I'm a mess," he began to allow himself to imagine dating a woman. As a leader of the singles volleyball league sponsored by his church, he had an opportunity to meet women. There was a quiet but friendly woman named Georgianna, who had a nice smile. His coughing and wheezing didn't put her off. She was attracted to this courageous man.

Georgianna had had an even more rugged life than Philip! She had been abused as a kid. She married to get away from home, but her husband turned out to be a felon who chased many skirts and eventually vanished with another man's wife. He filed for divorce, despite Georgianna's effort to maintain the marriage and her uncompromising veto of divorce. In the state they lived in, a petition for divorce is granted after one year, even if one party does not want it. After that, Georgianna's church ostracized her because she was a divorced woman. She raised three children without help from anyone, without welfare, working full time.

Philip and Georgianna fell in love and married. He now had one true friend. He accepted a job as a mathematics professor at a Christian school, Geneva College in Beaver Falls. The couple had no children other than the three from Georgianna's first marriage. The marriage was, with one exception, the best thing that ever happened to either of them. The one exception, according to Philip, was an even more excellent thing—both of them had been saved.

When Philip was forty-seven, some new medications were prescribed: Singulair (montelukast) and Pulmicort (budesonide). They revolutionized his life. He began to breathe as if he had no asthma. The peak airflow of his lungs doubled and became better than that of an average healthy person. For the first time in forty-five years, he could breathe through his nose. On the tennis court he excelled.

And so, because of advances in the science of medicine, Philip's story has an unexpected happy ending. At age fifty he has a good marriage and is a college professor of mathematics. He has friendly acquaintances throughout the faculty, but Georgianna is his only close friend. Every night he sleeps without coughing or wheezing and is no longer astonished to find that he is still alive at dawn.

Amazing Medicines

Philip's story illustrates that medical research and new drugs, such as beclomethasone, montelukast and budesonide, can actually give people new life. Because of medical research, Philip was able to have a sufficient supply of air for the first time in his life. Imagine, prior to the development of these medications, how many people like Philip suffered their entire lives and eventually died of suffocation!

Through my interviews I have found that the impact of conventional medicine is overwhelmingly positive. This message is the opposite of what I find in Dr. Andrew Weil's books (*Spontaneous Healing, Natural Health—Natural Medicine, Health and Healing*). Weil teaches that conventional medicine (also known as allopathic medicine) is dangerous and usually destructive. I have a lot of respect for naturopaths, and I think Weil gives some practical advice, such as taking charge of your own care. But I have found in my research that allopathic medicine is held in high regard by most of the sick people I interview. My difference of opinion with Dr. Weil reflects our different sampling methods. People seek Weil out because they are dissatisfied with allopathic medicine. Someone like Philip Holladay, who has success with allopathic medicine, is unlikely to seek treatment from Dr. Weil.

Strategy Sixteen: Keep Busy

If you are sick, everyday life can be a struggle. Sometimes it is easier to give up, accept defeat, and withdraw into your bedroom. This is a bad idea. If you live as a defeated, passive person, you will be unhappy. One of my patients tells me that at fibromyalgia support groups she meets people who have given up on life and become passive victims of the disease. Such an attitude allows the disease to become their dominant experience, eclipsing the nobility and dignity of life. Avoiding this mindset is the reason a job is valuable. Even a lousy job forces you to get out of bed and get to work, which is a positive thing if you are sickly. Keeping busy helps you to forget your troubles some of the time and enjoy the blessings that God gives all of us in such abundance.

The word *busy* needs to be defined in a realistic way. I will tell you four brief stories about people who keep busy.

Tom Whittaker was thirty-one years old when an out-of-control vehicle smashed into his car, leading to the amputation of his right leg below the knee. He loved hiking and returned to it with an artificial leg. Two years later he founded an organization called the Cooperative Wilderness Handicapped Outdoor Group. At age fifty he became the first person with an artificial leg ever to climb Mount Everest.

In chapter 2 I wrote about Jim Lubin, a quadriplegic due to a high spinal cord injury (C2). He has no control over his arms, legs, or trunk and is permanently dependent on a respirator. Because he was too disabled to do almost anything, he found rehab training depressing. About the only muscle Jim could control was his tongue and he thereby could control the direction of the airflow in his throat. A man named Denis Anson taught Jim how to use a device called a sip-and-puff interface. This is a small gadget attached to Jim's air tube that encodes an electronic signal, depending on which way the air is flowing in Jim's throat. This binary signal (zero or one) is fed into a computer and read by the computer as Morse code. Using this code Jim can type seventeen words per minute into the computer. With this ability he has developed an elaborate and magnificent Internet website (www.makoa.org).

Jim and I have corresponded by email. He tells me he spends nine hours a day working on his website and responding to email. Because of this activity, Jim finds his life rich and rewarding. He doesn't really consider himself disabled, because he has been able to work around the roadblock in his spinal cord.

Also in chapter 2 you read the story of Brooke Ellison, who was hit by an automobile when she was in the seventh grade. She ended up in the same shape as Jim Lubin—a quadriplegic and dependent on a respirator. Her tongue was the biggest muscle she could control. Brooke remained active by means of a device inserted in the roof of her mouth—a simple keyboard that could control a computer that allows her to communicate with the world around her and control an electric wheelchair. She was a brilliant student, graduating magna cum laude in May 2000 from Harvard University.

You might think that the worst thing that could happen to you would be to be paralyzed and on a respirator, like Jim or Brooke. But I'll tell you a worse story! There is something called the locked-in syndrome, which consists of a stroke so high in the brain stem that the person cannot even control his or her tongue. A person who is "locked in" is conscious, can see and hear, but the only way to get a message out to other people is via batting his or her eyelids. Such a person is taught to blink once if she or he wants to say yes, and twice if she or he wants to say no. This slow and laborious communication is the only way the locked-in person can communicate with other people.

So here's the story: A woman in her eighties was locked in. Her minister, while visiting, confided in her that he had so many prayer requests that he couldn't attend to them all. He asked for her help. She blinked once, agreeing to help. The minister went over the list of the members of their church who needed prayers. The locked-in woman started praying. This brought her a great sense of inner peace and satisfaction, especially when members of her church visited and commented on how her prayers had been answered. The locked-in woman lived only a few months, but during that time she kept busy with intercessory prayer, which brought her comfort, distraction from her imprisonment, and a sense of purpose.[7]

God created Adam and Eve in the image of God (Gen. 1:26–27). Theologians debate what aspect of humans constitutes the "image of God." One characteristic that is evident in the Bible is having dominion over the earth (Gen. 1:28–30; Ps. 8:4–8). Therefore it is reasonable that you should have dominion over your illness, rather than vice versa.

8

THE WISDOM OF CAREGIVERS

When we use the word *caregiver* inside the medical profession, we usually refer to those who are paid to take care of sick people, like nurses and allied health professionals. Often we overlook the person who gives the most care—the unpaid caregiver. The family members and neighbors who take care of sick people, making sure they have food to eat and driving them to the doctor's office, are often taken for granted in the medical world. Yet they have always been the backbone of medical care, more important than doctors or nurses. Today unpaid caregivers are becoming even more important as the number of people with chronic illnesses increases.

Who are the unpaid caregivers? Three-quarters of them are women, usually daughters or wives (figure 9), usually under the age of sixty-five. The average caregiver spends many hours per day giving care. Half of caregivers are employed; 40 percent of them are employed full-time.[1] But they are just barely able to juggle all their responsibilities. It is a challenge for them to get to work on time and to stay at work even when there is a crisis at home. They live a frantic lifestyle, often ignoring their own needs.[2]

Figure 9

Who Are the Unpaid Caregivers?

Females 72%   **Males 28%**

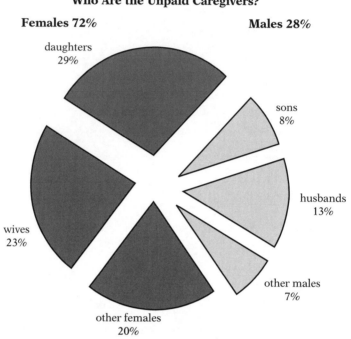

Data from Institute for Health and Aging, *Chronic Care in America* (Princeton, NJ: Robert Wood Johnson Foundation, 1996), 63

What is the economic value of the unpaid caregivers? In 1997 some economists estimated it to be 196 billion dollars in the United States, which dwarfs the amount of money our country spent on nursing homes (83 billion dollars) and home health aides (32 billion dollars) that year. In other words, the economic value of unpaid caregivers is far greater than the economic value of nursing homes, visiting nurses, and allied health professionals combined.[3]

Of course the needs and perspective of caregivers are different from the needs and perspective of sick people. For many of us, including caregivers, it is easy to focus on the sick people and forget about the caregivers, who tend to focus on the needs of the afflicted person and forget about themselves. They put their own needs dead last, as if they didn't matter.

Unfortunately, a crisis is brewing. There are fewer and fewer unpaid caregivers, just when the need for caregivers is increasing. In other words, the primary system for taking care of sick people is weakening and crumbling. There are four reasons for this:

1. Smaller family size. It is easier to care for a sick person in a family of eight than in a family of two.
2. Increased mobility. We often live hundreds of miles from our parents and siblings, so we cannot easily help when they get sick.
3. Fewer self-sacrificial people. The concept of self-sacrifice, central to caregiving, is often maligned in secular culture. Sometimes those who give their time so that someone else can live are spoken of negatively as "codependent" or "not taking care of their own needs." We drive our children to soccer practice and Little League but do nothing to teach them the value of taking care of someone else, even their parents when we get old.
4. Most women work outside the home. If three-quarters of caregivers are women, and most women work outside the home, there are fewer potential caregivers.

Many people have to quit their jobs to take care of a sick person. The two women you are about to meet gave up teaching careers to stay home as caregivers. As I tell you the story of two unpaid caregivers, I will be illustrating strategies seventeen and eighteen.

Strategy Seventeen: Take Pride in Your Work as a Caregiver

How can an unpaid caregiver, living in quiet obscurity and doing a difficult job, feel okay about her life? What is she accomplishing? Beth Brown believes she is doing the assignment God entrusted to her, taking care of her husband after his stroke. She radiates a tranquil joy, despite a burden that might have crushed someone else.

Don Brown was a professor of educational psychology at the University of Colorado. He had a quick mind, was highly published, had a vast vita, and was involved in many projects, such as teaching reading and literacy to prisoners and inner-city adults.

When Don was thirty-eight years old, his first wife, Billie, died suddenly of a brain aneurysm, leaving him with five children to raise (Rick, Sharon, Steve, Kayleen, and David).

Beth Hollenbach, a twenty-year-old woman who lived across the street, took an interest in the kids because they were motherless. Well, one thing led to another, namely to Don and Beth getting married. Soon Beth gave birth to twins, Amy and April, and then for thirty years Don and Beth enjoyed a rich and rewarding family life and companionship, shared exciting conversation and dreams. Beth grew in the marriage, went through graduate school, and became a professor of education at Denver Seminary.

In chapter 4 I pointed out that the risk of illness increases with age (see figure 2). Don is nearly twenty years older than Beth and therefore is at greater risk of illness than she. When Don was sixty-eight years old, he had prostate cancer for which surgery was recommended. It was supposed to be a low-risk, routine surgery, and indeed it cured the cancer.

"You sign these consent forms for surgery," Beth says, "but you don't really know what you are getting into."

The day after the surgery a blood clot traveled to Don's brain and caused a bilateral thalamic stroke. Strokes of this kind are rare. When they do occur, they usually cause enormous pain, because the thalamus regulates pain signals from all over the body. Don had no pain. He was unconscious and in the intensive care unit for weeks. Nine weeks later he left the hospital for a five-week stay in a nursing home. Then he came home to Beth, a changed man. At that time Beth was fifty-one years old and their twin girls were twenty-nine.

Because of the stroke, Don lost his mental acuity. His recent memory was shot. He was so weak that he couldn't get out of bed or stand. With physical therapy he learned to stand and walk with a walker. After months of occupational therapy, he learned how to dress himself. After four years Beth began to realize that Don's quick mind wasn't coming back.

"He is still very intelligent in some areas," she says, "but slow in others. He has trouble learning new tasks. For example, I tried for a long time to teach him how to use a credit card at the gas pump. He just couldn't do it. So I got out and put in the card while he removed the gas cap and pumped the gas. He took pleasure in helping.

"When you have lots of losses," says Beth, "you can either dwell on the losses or accept them and try to move on with whatever life is now possible. I've found three Fs that allowed me to remain cheerful despite my husband's stroke: family, friends, and faith. I've gotten much closer to the Lord because of Don's condition. So you could say, 'Isn't it worth it to get this close to the Lord?' I would reply, 'Maybe! But, come on! Let's get real! If I had the opportunity to have the old Don back, I would jump at it.'"

Now Beth spends most of her time sitting quietly at home with her husband. Because he tires so easily, morning is Don's best time of day. As the day progresses, he fades. "I try to engage him in conversation in the morning," Beth says. "He cherishes our time together and so do I.

"There isn't a day that goes by," Beth continues, "that I don't miss my husband as he used to be—vital, energetic, and enthusiastic! I miss the family life we had, our dreams, and all of that. For the most part I have grieved that loss. There are still moments when grief grabs me by surprise and washes over me, but I don't stay there long."

Many people are uncertain at times how God wants them to live. But Beth trusts God for his direction. She says, "We search the mind of God to know what his will would be for this season of our lives."

When it comes to taking care of Don, Beth is facing a difficult assignment, but she has no doubt about God's will. "My present call is clear," Beth continues. "Take care of Don and do it with my whole heart! Joy comes from simply being obedient to the call of God. I truly delight in caring for Don. I'm doing what God asked me to do and I'm doing it with enthusiasm. This private ministry is fulfilling because I know that God smiles on me. Don is sweet and appreciative, which makes caring for him all the easier.

"I finally adjusted to the huge change in my life, from the dynamic of teaching in a lively classroom to my new quiet life. I used to be so extroverted that being confined at home, especially during the first year, nearly killed me. Now I would describe myself as content. I take pleasure in taking care of Don, running our household, and staying busy. I stay busy by being a good mother to my adult children, a fun grandma, and a good friend. When I'm home, I keep the house clean, prepare meals, and pay the bills.

"During the afternoon, when Don naps, I usually quilt," Beth continues. "Quilting gives me real pleasure and a sense of accomplishment. I enjoy working with fabric, color, and design. It is an opportunity to create something for people I love. I have something to show for my time at the end, but the quiet activity is a blessing in itself. It helps me to slow down and enjoy the present moment."

I ask Beth how it feels to lose her teaching career. She corrects me, saying that she is *still* teaching! "Don and I teach with our day-to-day lives how to live with loss in a way that glorifies God. Our children, grandchildren, friends, and others are watching us adjust to multiple losses and yet still live gratefully, with genuine joy, and with confidence in the goodness of God. He is so good!

"At my daughters' insistence," Beth says, "I take two respite trips a year. They work out who will stay with their dad while I'm gone. Last year Amy went to Baltimore with me to visit my brother, and April and I took a trip to Southern California for a long weekend at the beach, Disneyland, art galleries, and so on. This year I'm planning to visit my college roommate and I don't know what else. These trips give me something to look forward to for months!"

Beth describes something that is crucial for caregivers—taking some time off. But this is possible only when someone else takes over the responsibility to provide respite care.

"Where is God in all this?" Beth asks. "Everywhere! In those early months of despair, I rose early in the morning, read the Word, and wept. I prayed the Psalms, which was the most important help of all. God healed me, strengthened me, and has been my 'husband.'

"Don has made remarkable progress," Beth continues. "Today he gets up, showers and dresses, and makes our breakfast! He brings in the morning paper. After breakfast I have Don read to me from a devotional book and then we journal. I started this practice with him so that his word-finding skills would improve and so that I could get some daily insight into what he was thinking and feeling. After we journal, we read each other's entries out loud and talk about what we've written. Then we pray. This can last until ten in the morning. A sweet time!"

Beth can now leave Don at home alone for an hour or two. Their daughter Kayleen provided a cell phone so that Beth can stay in touch with Don when she's out. He can answer the phone and has learned to write down a phone message. He reads the paper, rides his stationary bike six miles a day five days a week, follows the Bronco football games, and writes family memoirs on his computer.

I asked Beth what advice she would give to a woman whose husband just suffered a stroke.

"I wouldn't give a woman any advice one month after her husband's stroke," she replied. "What could be said that would help? Nothing could have eased my grief at that moment. When well-meaning people shared their insights with me at that time, I quickly understood that they had no idea how I felt or the depth of my grief and confusion. The friends that most helped were the ones who simply hung in there with me, those who stayed close."

It's important to understand what Beth has said. A good friend to a caregiver or sick person is one who is loyal and available over the long haul. Many friends will be there at first, but their enthusiasm fades as the true meaning of the word *chronic* becomes clear, namely, long-long-long-term.

Beth continues, "I searched for help in written form at the time of Don's stroke. I needed medical information so that I could begin to understand what was happening to him and what our future might be. My children searched the Internet, and I purchased a few books about stroke and rehabilitation. What would have helped would have been the stories of other women whose husbands had strokes and how they felt and how their stories progressed.

"I believe in 'normalizing' the pain and confusion and, above all, in giving hope, hope that this despair will ease with time and that adjustments can be made, hope that someday you will know joy again, hope that heaven awaits where there will be no more sorrow or tears."

Self-Respect

Strategy seventeen is "Take pride in your work as a caregiver." Beth dislikes the word *pride*. As a devout Christian, Beth thinks of pride as a negative word, a sin, the opposite of how a Christian ought to be. She and I debate whether *pride* can sometimes be a positive word. I use *pride* in a positive sense, meaning a sense of one's own proper dignity or value; self-respect. According to the dictionary, it also conveys a sense of "pleasure or satisfaction taken in an achievement." When I use the word *pride*, I am referring to the nobility of the human spirit. The more adverse the circumstances on the battlefield of health, the more some warriors stand out as majestic and courageous, the way a black velvet background makes a diamond sparkle brighter in a jewelry store window.

Instead of the word *pride*, if I used the term *self-respect*, Beth would be more comfortable, because she would agree that it is okay for a caregiver to feel self-respect. Beth finds satisfaction in knowing that her work is valuable and valued. I could say it this way: Beth takes comfort in her quiet and private ministry of caregiving, knowing that she is faithful to the assignment that God has given her, namely taking care of Don.

It might be hard for someone who is not carrying a heavy burden to appreciate what I am talking about. Both Beth Brown and Charlene Stephens (whose story follows) are taking care of someone with brain damage. There is a sense in which both women know that as caregivers they are doing about as good a job as anyone could do. They are obedient to God. It is reasonable under such circumstances that they should take comfort in doing a difficult job well.

The attitude of the sick person makes all the difference in caregiving. Some caregivers live with a sick person who is grumpy or self-destructive, for example refusing to adhere to the diet or not following the doctor's orders. That makes caregiving onerous and difficult. Carol Levine, for example, wrote a heartbreaking essay in the *New England Journal of Medicine* about her tragic life taking care of an irritable husband who had had a stroke.[4] Fortunately Don is not like that. As Beth says, it is Don's cooperation and appreciation that makes her task pleasant.

Part of what this means is that someone who is stricken, who depends on other people for survival, has a calling in life, namely to be pleasant and to make the caregiver's task a blessing. Sick people who pray for their caregivers are more likely to smile and give cheerful nonverbal signals when the caregiver is nearby.

Epilogue

It has been thirty months since I interviewed Beth Brown and wrote her story. During that time she and Don moved to Evans, Colorado, to be closer to their daughter Amy. This resulted in a vast improvement in Beth's quality of life. To begin with, her grandchildren bring sunshine into her life, and she laughs now when she talks with me on the phone. Rev. Doug Brown invited Beth to join the staff of the First United Presbyterian Church in Greeley, teaching ten hours a week on a schedule that allows her to take care of Don. So now Beth feels she's engaged with the wider world again, no longer isolated at home, and using her teaching skills. For the last nine months she has blossomed.

Strategy Eighteen: Enjoy the Blessings

Charlene Stephens of Woodbury, Connecticut, has a daughter named Carla who is sixteen years old. Carla has never learned to stand or walk. She has no language, cannot feed herself, has a mental age of less than one year, and is unable to control her urine or bowels. She lives in a wheelchair or bed and must be watched constantly for the onset of uncontrollable seizures.

Carla was normal at birth and for her first five months. Then she began to lapse into states of being unresponsive. The doctors could not decide what was wrong. It turned out that Carla was having absence seizures. These were epileptic seizures but were evident only in Carla's unresponsiveness. Doctors are unsure about the cause of the seizures, but it may have been a bad reaction to her second DPT vaccination. That was inferred from the timing of their onset.

The problem with the seizures became deadly serious when Carla was eleven months old and had a second MMR vaccination. After that she developed grand mal seizures that wouldn't stop. She was taken by ambulance to the emergency room for treatment. During the ambulance ride, she stopped breathing and was resuscitated. This was the beginning of sixteen hospitalizations. With a desperately ill child, Charlene was frantic when the doctors were unable to reach an agreement about what was the cause or prognosis. One doctor told Charlene, "She will be a basket case." The next said, "Carla will be completely normal." Another predicted: "She will be confined to a wheelchair."

"At first the people in my church prayed for Carla to be healed," Charlene said. "I believe in miraculous healing, in God's restorative powers. But somehow I knew that Carla wasn't going to be healed. So these prayers disturbed me. As long as I prayed for healing, or the people around me were praying for it, that was an obstacle that distracted me. Those prayers prevented me from doing what I needed to do. They were a barrier between my child and me. I needed to mourn for the healthy child, to let go of that dream and let that imaginary child die. The prayers for healing just got in the way, encouraging me to withdraw emotionally from Carla as she actually was and keep my hopes invested in the imaginary Carla that would never be. My mother stepped in and helped me take care of Carla in the beginning, because I withdrew from her. Externally I took care of her as I needed to do, but I drew back and was disengaged, aloof, and emotionally distant.

"Eventually I learned a better kind of prayer. I prayed that I would be able to accept Carla as she is and would be given the strength to be the best parent that I could be. That was a much better way to pray. And that prayer was answered."

Charlene left the church that was insisting on healing prayer and joined another church that was more accepting of the chronic condition. This shows the problem with healing prayer, namely that God often answers such prayer with a no, but the people praying refuse to accept God's answer.

"People are afraid of Carla," Charlene continues. "Even people at my new church are afraid. They don't want to get near her because they don't know what to say or do. They feel awkward. We used to take Carla to church and leave her in the nursery while Bill and I would worship, but we no longer do that. It isn't appropriate. It is asking too much of the people who run the nursery."

At first, it was a disappointment to have a child who was so different from the one for whom Charlene planned, hoped, and prepared. It was also disappointing to have to give up her job. Prior to Carla's birth, Charlene had taught English and photojournalism in the public schools. But with Carla's needs, it was impossible to continue working away from home. Now Charlene stays home most of the time.

That's true of many caregivers—they spend many silent hours inside a house. They are the unsung heroes.

By age seven Carla's seizures became more frequent, complex, and difficult to treat. Medications would work for a few years then stop working. As far as Charlene knows, her daughter would have been mentally normal except for the damage caused by the seizures. As it is, Carla is profoundly mentally retarded.

"You never know for sure," says Charlene. "Perhaps there was something wrong from the beginning and we didn't notice it. But we think her retardation is caused by brain damage due to prolonged seizures."

I asked Charlene if she ever considered allowing the seizures to go untreated, so that Carla would die and go to Jesus.

"I have never considered not treating Carla's seizures," Charlene replied. "I don't feel that I have the right to determine Carla's existence. I feel very strongly that I have been given the capability and the wherewithal to care for her and I will do so as long as I am able. She is, to the best of my ability to perceive, happy and content.

"If Carla had been in an institution she would be dead by now," Charlene says.

It is only because of the careful attention of a devoted mother that this child survived. When Carla's seizures began, Charlene started keeping an elaborate journal, charting everything about Carla, from her diet to body temperature to the nuances of behavior. Only after months of careful observations did Charlene discover that the seizures were triggered by small changes in temperature, such as would be caused by an ear infection raising body temperature or an air-conditioned grocery store lowering Carla's body temperature. Since these seizures were often unresponsive to medication, such observation about how to avoid the seizures was lifesaving. Such observations would never have been made in an institution, and Carla would have died.

"I am still angry," Charlene admits. "I'm not angry at anyone. I'm angry that things turned out this way."

Yet it is not anger that comes through when I talk with Charlene. There is an astonishing gladness and enjoyment of life that is the dominant theme. This woman finds every day delightful.

"It is no use dwelling on the things we can't do because of Carla," Charlene says. "What we choose to focus on is that we do things differently because of Carla."

When I visited their house, I found that Carla and Charlene have rich interactions in terms of facial expression, tone of voice, and body language.

"Carla is easy to be with and to love," Charlene says. "She enjoys snuggles and kisses and having her back rubbed. Being with Carla is like being with an infant who has not yet learned how to manipulate others. She will not throw a tantrum because you are doing something she doesn't want to do. Sometimes she gets quiet, and like many nonverbal children, she is hard to read at those times. You have to be connected to her so you can be aware of small behaviors that give you a clue as to what is going on when she is uncommunicative.

"Carla doesn't need to be entertained," Charlene continues. "She loves listening to music." There is usually music playing in Charlene's house. And Carla likes the sound of people's voices. If there is a basketball or baseball game on TV, she loves hearing that. She likes going out for rides in the car or going through shopping malls, providing it is not too crowded or noisy. If she is in her wheelchair, where she feels safe, she enjoys being outside.

Over the years, as Carla has grown in size, it has become increasingly difficult to care for her. Charlene can still lift Carla from the wheelchair to the car. But the child's bedroom is upstairs, and she now weighs too much for Charlene to carry her up, so Bill does that.

As Carla gets older, people are less accepting of her handicap. If a five-year-old acts like an infant, the public will accept that, but not if a sixteen-year-old does so. There is too much disparity between what people expect and how this adolescent behaves. Charlene can't take Carla to a restaurant because her behavior would be inappropriate. You wouldn't take an infant into a movie theater. Similarly, you can't take Carla to the movies either. So as Carla gets older, the problems increase and tend to keep Charlene and Bill at home most of the time.

When Gina, Carla's sister, was younger and lived at home, Bill and Charlene had the freedom to go out to a movie from time to time. But now that Gina is away at college, it is no longer realistic to spend an evening away from Carla. Ordinary babysitters are not prepared to take care of someone who might have uncontrollable seizures. Agencies can provide a trained person to care for Carla for an evening, but then Bill and Charlene would spend one hundred dollars on babysitting simply to go out and watch a movie. They don't think it's worth it.

Four-and-a-half days a week, from 8:00 A.M. to 2:30 P.M., Carla goes to a state-funded school called Aces Village School. With the commuting time in the school van, she is gone from 7:30 A.M. till 3:30 P.M. The school has nurses and personnel who are trained to deal with Carla. Having this amount of time away from Carla has allowed Charlene and Bill to avoid burnout.

Respite care is crucial if the caregiver is to maintain her or his morale. More respite programs are needed, as fewer full-time caregivers are available. Unfortunately, various laws, insurance regulations, and bureaucratic restrictions often prevent respite programs from operating. For example, a hospital near me tried to open some respite beds to meet the great need. Before ever opening a single bed, they were overwhelmed with hassles over regulations and laws, insurance restrictions, and the nature of their charter and were never able to offer respite care. We as a society must be careful to support and encourage our unpaid caregivers. They are a precious resource.

Charlene has followed strategy seventeen and takes pride in how she and Bill have cared for Carla. They have been excellent parents.

Charlene admits that she is haunted by the question of what will happen to Carla when they are no longer around to take care of her. "Who will care about her and be concerned about the day-to-day care responsibilities?" she asks. "There is no answer. But maybe the answer is—I just don't know if anyone will. Perhaps her sister will, but that is a great burden to place on Gina's shoulders. That is a very painful thought—of Carla being uncared for and unloved. It is almost something that I cannot stand to think about—I put it out of my mind almost immediately when it surfaces."

Charlene and Bill have turned a hobby into a cottage industry. They buy, sell, and repair antique dolls. Specifically, they work with antique bisque dolls that were made in Germany or France from 1870 to 1930 and with the furniture and clothing for such dolls. Charlene is a superb artist. She is able to repair damaged ceramic and restore ancient clothing. Bill took early retirement from his teaching job. During my interview with Charlene, Bill was out at a doll auction. The couple's website is www.vintagevignettes.com.

Charlene also sculpts. She makes Santa Claus dolls in exactly the style of the antique dolls, with ceramic bodies, glass eyes, and clothing made in the way that doll clothes were made a century ago. Charlene's dolls, ranging from five inches to thirty-six inches tall, are for sale in the Pierre Hotel in Manhattan, and in the Mayflower Inn in Washington Depot, Connecticut.

Charlene counts her blessings. "I love my house," she says. "I enjoy living every day. By this I mean that every morning I wake up looking forward to the day. I don't deny that Carla is work, more work than other sixteen-year-old daughters. But I choose not to dwell on that. This ability to remain positive comes from spiritual grounding. It is also a personality trait. My self-esteem is secure, so I don't need feedback from my daughter to make me feel I am okay.

"I come from a heritage of strong women. My mother's mother survived the unexpected and tragic deaths of four husbands. She had an indomitable spirit. She could have been dragged down by so much tragedy, losing people she loved to car accidents, illness, and even murder. But she chose joy. My grandmother was the happiest person I ever knew.

"The life trip we all plan for and fully expect is sometimes detoured for unexplained reasons," Charlene summarizes. "We can either accept that detour, however unfair it may be, and enjoy the unexpected and very different sights, or we can rail against our assignment in life, making our lives a long journey of frustration and unfulfilled hopes. I have chosen to accept my change of itinerary, with God's help, and have found unexpected joy in that choice.

"I can't stand it when Christians say that everything is perfect in their lives and that they wouldn't want God to change a single thing. The truth is that if I could have Carla restored to normal, I would do it in a heartbeat. I don't like things the way they are, but I have chosen to accept them. People have no idea what our life has been like. That's because no two disabilities are the same. Not even two children with seizures are the same."

At the time of our interview Charlene was fifty-one and Bill fifty-three years old. Gina, age nineteen, came home for the Christmas holidays, which allowed the extra luxury of Bill and Charlene being able to go out for an evening at the movies. Basically, they feel that life is good. It is full of blessings.

Since I interviewed Charlene Stephens thirty months ago, Carla's condition has not changed. During that thirty months, Charlene made the decision to begin teaching four or five classes at two local colleges while Carla is cared for by others. There is more laughter in Charlene's voice today than there was when I interviewed her initially. It seems to be a breath of fresh air for her to be working part-time outside the house.

Charlene is a good example of someone living by strategy eighteen: Enjoy the blessings. She has taken life as it has come to her and is finding joy and blessings even in her difficult situation.

Self-Sacrifice

Jesus said, "Greater love has no one than this, that he lay down his life for his friends" (John 15:13). Both Beth and Charlene have been sacrificing their lives to take care of someone else. While doing so, they both manage to keep a smile on their faces. Beth recognizes that she is doing the job that God assigned to her. Charlene enjoys the unexpected blessings that God has given in caring for her handicapped daughter, even though she would prefer, of course, to have a healthy child.

As I said earlier, a crucial need today is for volunteers who will meet some of the needs of caregivers like Beth and Charlene. Jesus set the example by washing the disciples' feet. But few churches today wash the feet of the unpaid caregivers who often can't get away long enough to go to church. Mostly we can care for caregivers by befriending them, spending time with them, and providing respite care. But there are other things that could be done to help.

I recommend that caregivers take courses from the University without Walls, which is a teleconference program offering courses and workshops via the telephone to people who are homebound.[5] The discussions in this University are held by conference call, so that caregivers can stay at home. It is an excellent way to expand their horizons, stimulate their mind, perhaps even get a degree.

In any discussion of chronic illness, it is easy to focus on the suffering of the sick person, while failing to notice the problems of the healthy caregiver—they carry a heavy burden, and most suffer as a result. It's as though they are incarcerated in a frenetic lifestyle. Often there is a syndrome of what might be called overfunctioning, like an engine that is running at 110 percent of its maximum capacity. There is what might be called overcompetence—the caregiver juggles full-time employment, running the household, caring for the sick person, and doing it all well with insufficient sleep and no days off! Unless someone else steps in to provide respite care, there are no days free of responsibility. If you think of Charlene, what makes her life tolerable is that Carla goes to school four-and-a-half days a week. But, as I said, many caregivers of Alzheimer's sufferers have no respite at all. Some caregivers have not had a single day off in five years.

I am not saying this picture fits all caregivers, but there is a tendency among many caregivers toward extreme self-sacrifice. Sometimes such people are accused of failing to take care of their own needs. Self-sacrifice used to be considered a virtue, but today the term is often used as an accusation, as if it implies masochism. Such accusations need to be cushioned with realism. When the only alternative is abandoning the sick person, the caregiver has little choice.

As the tide of chronic illness rises, and as the population ages, leading to a doubling of the number of people with Alzheimer's disease, there will be an increasing need for unpaid caregivers. Yet simultaneously there is a decreasing supply. This is a crisis throughout the world, yet public policy and churches are mostly ignoring it.

You don't have to be featured on the front page of the newspaper to know that you are doing something important. Many caregivers, such as Beth Brown and Charlene Stephens, live in quiet obscurity, but they understand that they are doing a praiseworthy job taking care of someone who could not survive on his or her own.

I once treated a woman who took care of her elderly and sickly parents. She said, "I know that when I get to heaven, Jesus will meet me at the pearly gates and say, 'Well done, good and faithful servant!'" (see Matt. 25:21, 23).

9

FROM DISABLED TO IS ABLE

Imagine, if you will, that all around you are normal couples your age, pursuing their careers, with enough time, money, and energy to enjoy a decent lifestyle, own houses, raise children, and go on vacations. But your spouse, whom you love dearly, suffers from a chronic illness that causes such agony that it eclipses all other goals and imposes a demand that you must leave no stone unturned in a quest for relief from the pain.

Imagine that you are an optimist. You hope that just around the corner there is some untried treatment that promises to release your spouse from the jaws of the disease that is chewing her or him up. Conventional approaches to medicine have failed, so you turn to Complementary and Alternative Medical treatments that are expensive and not covered by health insurance. You have already decided to abandon your career, because of financial reasons, and have turned to another, more lucrative career that might someday provide enough money and health insurance to escape the unending crush of medical bills. Meanwhile, all your time, money, and energy are invested in trying to solve or at least endure this endless siege.

Things look bleak. Both you and your spouse have had to give up your careers, you are penniless, and the prospect of ever owning a house or affording a vacation is remote.

If you were in such a situation, how would you avoid feeling bitter? Randy John's answer to that question is that you must begin by avoiding any comparison of your life with the lives of other couples.

But, you might ask, How can I do that? It is only natural to compare how my spouse and I are doing with our peer group!

You have learned to shun such comparisons because they are so painful. Furthermore, many of your peers have rejected you. You and your spouse are like social outcasts, so it is easier than you might expect to avoid such comparisons, because the people you would have thought were in your peer group have made it clear that you are unacceptable as a peer.

It is a lonely business, being the spouse of someone with a chronic disease. Your partner is often lonely, so you tend to want to stay home to provide companionship. Not only must you shoulder the burden of caring for your partner, but you must do so in isolation. Other people, even your family, cannot understand what you are going through. It is as if you were from another planet, an alien, perhaps a leper. Other people cannot or choose not to empathize with you. If your spouse would either die or recover, then you would be welcomed back into the company of human society.

It is far more acceptable in America to be dying of cancer than failing to die from a persistent illness. Apparently a life sentence is worse than a death sentence. People around you have no experience that allows them to understand what it means to remain sickly with an invisible disability, year in and year out.

Invisible disabilities are worse than visible ones.[1] A friend of Randy's describes people with invisible disabilities:

> Their suffering is masked by a healthy appearance. They are not in wheelchairs and do not use canes. Yet their pain and debility is real and chronic. They have "invisible disabilities." It may be the soul-sapping fatigue, environmental sensitivity, and chronic pain of fibromyalgia, or lupus, or Lyme disease, or multiple sclerosis. These souls suffer not only from their diseases but often from the uninformed and hurtful reactions of others. . . . When someone looks healthy, we are tempted to

tell them to "just buck up" and do what we think they should do. Those with invisible disabilities are often expected to do what is beyond them. We would never tell someone who uses a cane to run a marathon, but just going to the store may be a marathon for someone with lupus.[2]

Randy John married Susan McCullagh when he was twenty-seven and she was twenty-six. They were both healthy and athletic and had an enjoyable life together. Gymnastics and dance were the essence of who Susan was. She excelled in track in high school. Susan loved to swim and hike with Randy. Sooner or later they planned to have children or adopt. At Denver Seminary he studied theology. His career goal was to be ordained, plant new churches, and spread the gospel. She had an undergraduate degree in fine arts. At seminary Susan studied counseling. As I write this, they have been married twelve-and-a-half years. It is a good marriage.

Unfortunately Susan slowly began to develop health problems. She had many pains. Her muscles and joints ached throughout her body. During the second half of her menstrual cycle, she had pelvic pain, depression, and irritability. She was increasingly exhausted for no apparent reason. These problems got insidiously worse over the years. Chemicals in the environment, such as paint fumes, perfumes, or automobile exhaust, aggravated Susan's symptoms. The couple turned to physicians for help, but these mysterious problems often eluded medical treatment. Seven years ago a doctor diagnosed Susan as having fibromyalgia with chronic fatigue syndrome, as well as a severe case of premenstrual syndrome (PMS). Standard therapies, such as antidepressant medication, were tried but didn't help. As Susan's body became increasingly reactive to hormones and environmental chemicals, she also became more susceptible to the side effects of medicines. At the present time there are few medicines that she can tolerate, and of those almost none has a positive effect.

Susan's lifestyle has been eroded by these illnesses. She is so often weak and depressed that she can no longer work. Pain emerged as the primary culprit. If pain is ranked on a scale from one to ten (with ten being the worst pain imaginable), Susan's baseline on her good days is five or six. The ache is spread diffusely throughout her muscles and joints, especially her neck, back, and shoulders. She has fewer than twelve good days per month. Her body is especially sensitive to progesterone, the natural hormone of the second half of a menstrual cycle. During that half of her cycle, Susan develops agonizing pelvic pain, especially on the left side. This ranks nine or ten on the pain scale. It is so torturous that it eclipses the other pains, which are still present. Along with this come storm clouds of despair and agitation that overshadow Susan's normally sunny disposition. She is a trained mental health professional, well aware of what is happening, but she cannot prevent herself from being sucked into the vortex of agony.

When local physicians failed to provide relief, the couple, at great expense, sought out experts in distant states and at leading medical centers. They prayed constantly for God's guidance and comfort, for God to heal, and for the strength to endure another day. One alternative care physician gave Susan some medicine that helped decrease the mental and emotional volatility of PMS, but the doctor's attitude was so obnoxious that they decided not to go back. They turned to acupuncture and a variety of Complementary and Alternative Medical treatments, some of which provided moderate relief, but after a while even those failed. When I interviewed Randy, he and Susan were on the brink of deciding in favor of a hysterectomy, even though they were childless. They still looked forward to adopting from abroad, perhaps a group of siblings.

Randy John was a full-time student in an arduous doctoral program when I interviewed him. There was shopping, cooking, housework to be attended to on the days when Susan was incapacitated. Although his desire was to become a minister, he heard the Lord calling him in a different direction. Let's face it, on average, clergy are poorly paid and have lousy health insurance. This is especially true of ministers who specialize in planting new churches as Randy had wished to do. Clergy tend to work more than a forty-hour week and therefore are less available at home. Randy's marital responsibilities made it unrealistic for him to pursue ordination.

He has chosen to become a chiropractor. Randy has his own chronic illness, Ménière's syndrome, and his condition has improved through the care of a chiropractor. If he goes several months without a chiropractic adjustment, he is plagued with ringing in his ears and dizziness.

At the time of our interview, Randy and Susan were living in Romulus, New York, while he was a student at the New York Chiropractic College in Seneca Falls. Subsequently they moved to the town of

Wareham in Massachusetts where Randy will practice as a chiropractor. Perhaps, sometime down the road, Randy hopes that the Lord
will call him back into the ministry.

Susan remains a creative, courageous, and delightful woman. She
is highly intelligent and well read. She and Randy can dialogue on
a multitude of different levels. Whereas Randy is an introvert who
has learned to be extroverted, Susan is naturally extroverted, spontaneous, and witty. Her core personality is still there, despite being
whittled down by the illness. Like Randy she tries to find hope, often
through prayer and sticking close to God. The couple enjoys music
and singing. Sometimes they lead worship services together. Susan
is trying, when she has enough energy, to get back into her artwork,
using acrylic paints and watercolors. She is an exceptional artist. In all
arenas Susan's creativity is apparent, especially in the way she makes
simple things special and makes their home attractive. Currently she
is putting together a book of art and poetry by people with chronic
illnesses, with the title "Tears of Tenacity."

Strategy Nineteen: Suffer Fools Lightly

People with invisible disabilities suffer twice. Their disability causes
suffering as do the unsympathetic people who misunderstand their
chronic condition. "What is wrong with you?" they ask. "Why don't
you come out of your house and join the human race, have some
fun, get a life, let yourself be lighthearted for a change? Why do you
choose to wallow in your misery?" Since there is no wheelchair, they
assume there is no obstacle.

Someone once said, "Anyone who can turn on a radio thinks he or
she understands music." Randy John says, "Anyone who has had a
headache thinks he or she understands chronic pain, but they don't.
When you are a chronic pain sufferer, you cannot simply choose to
come out of your house and join the human race, have some fun, or
get a life, as people advise. It is not that we choose to wallow in our
misery. Rather, it is that the distress that grips my wife rarely allows
her any respite from harassment."

Randy's comments illustrate strategy nineteen: Suffer fools lightly.
The term *fools* refers to the healthy people who are fair-weather

friends. All too often they are spouses who divorce a sick partner, pretending they never said the words "in sickness and in health" in the marriage vows.

Randy and Susan have been rejected by friends and they suffer social isolation because of Susan's chronic condition. Today people expect friends to do things with them. Friendship is usually activity oriented. "Let's go for a walk . . . play golf . . . meet for coffee or go shopping." Furthermore, there is usually an expectation that you will be able to make plans and hold to them.

Now consider what these requirements are like for people like Randy and Susan. To begin with, you can forget about being activity oriented. Susan is often too physically and emotionally depleted to leave the apartment. So chances are you wouldn't even meet her in the first place, so it would never occur to you to befriend her—out of sight, out of mind.

Many sick people cannot make future plans. They have no idea how they will feel tomorrow or next week. The best they can do is make tentative plans. A chronically ill person might have to say, "If I feel better than usual, then we might be lucky and be able to get together for lunch tomorrow, assuming I am not nauseated." When someone who is chronically ill phones to cancel a lunch date, what does that mean? Many healthy people take it personally. *She doesn't like me,* they assume. They get angry, hurt, or distant. Most often they drop the ill person as a friend. It never occurs to them (or they don't believe) that he or she phoned to cancel because the pain and fatigue were overwhelming. It doesn't occur to healthy people that even making a phone call may take Herculean strength and determination, that life is like swimming upstream in white-water rapids. These obstacles make maintaining friendships difficult.

Consider the following paragraph from Patricia Fennell's book *The Chronic Illness Workbook*:

> "I was talking on the phone with Cindy," Joan said, "and she was tell-ing me about the new man in her life and about how they were trying to blend their work styles and homes and furniture and all. Then she asked me about my life. I didn't know what to say. Finally I said that I didn't really want to lay all my symptoms on her. But as a matter of fact, I was thinking about how I had to choose between washing my hair or

going to the store. I didn't have enough energy to do both. Still, I'd been able to do a little picking up, and I thought that showed progress. She interrupted me and what she said . . . shocked me. She said, 'It's like the Joan I knew is dead. I don't recognize you anymore. It's like you're a completely different person.'"[3]

If you want to understand sick people, you have to learn to think in terms of poverty of resources. It's like the energy crisis. American society consumes three times more energy than any other nation. We take for granted our ability to use electricity and gasoline to accomplish our goals. But now shift your viewpoint and think of a rural village in a developing nation with scant energy, where people walk instead of using cars and hand-pump their water from a village well. Life is slower. Productivity is lower. The goals of life are modest, focused more on surviving until tomorrow. This is the type of shift that must occur in your thinking if you want to understand chronic illness.

People with disabilities tend to be more socially isolated than those without disabilities. They are twice as likely to live alone, much less likely to socialize with other people, and less likely to see a movie, concert, or sporting event. They are even less likely to go to a grocery store.[4]

The bottom line is, unless you are interested in seeking out disabled people and spending time with them at their convenience, you are likely to have a list of friends that includes few people with debilitating illnesses. Now this story has come full circle. That is where we began, with the isolation of Randy and Susan from those people who had previously been their peer group. When I said earlier that other people have rejected this couple because of illness, chances are most readers were puzzled. But now it may be easier to understand. Randy and Susan simply don't fit into the television image of the American lifestyle. To think that there could be so much suffering so close to home is painful. Most Americans would rather not think about it. It is too threatening—it might happen to them as well.

If a person has cancer and is going to die, that is respectable because the time of suffering is limited. We applaud the heroism of someone dying of cancer. We send flowers and cards and we visit, knowing that soon this misery will end. But how do we relate to people who are serving a life sentence of debilitating illness? They make healthy people feel awkward. What can you talk about? Chronically ill people are misfits in America. And often we turn our back on them.

Why is it so hard for us to accept people like Susan and Randy? Their potential friends seem to think that Susan can just get over her ailment and act like a normal person. Primarily there is a failure of imagination. It's hard to imagine that if Susan goes out in public, it will take every ounce of energy she can muster. If you think about it, what sort of shape do you think Susan would be in while she is out of the house? Would you expect her to be smiling, bubbling with laughter, effervescent, and high-spirited? Probably not! Probably she would be hanging on by her fingertips, drained of energy.

Someone who barely knows Susan, say another woman at church, might see Susan as sluggish, barely reacting to her environment. Her sentences are short. She doesn't initiate conversation. Rapidly the other woman arrives at the incorrect conclusion that Susan is aloof and unfriendly. The idea that sluggishness reflects illness never crosses the other woman's mind. This is what I mean by a failure of imagination. It is difficult to imagine how grim life is for someone with a debilitating illness if you don't see a wheelchair and you don't stop to ask the sick person what it is like getting out of the apartment for the first time in a week. In this respect, invisible disabilities are twice as bad as visible ones.

There are other obstacles that prevent us from opening ourselves up to the Susans of this world. We Americans are a hurried people. We drive in the fast lane. Life is a whirlwind. There is barely time to think. Sometimes this frantic pace is worse inside churches, with meetings seven evenings a week. It is virtually impossible for someone who is frenetic to relate to someone who is debilitated. The conflict is in terms of the pace of life. It is too wide a chasm to bridge. If you want to have a meaningful conversation with someone who is depleted, it takes time. You have to sit down, wait, talk patiently, listen slowly, tolerate silence, allow the other person to catch his or her breath. If you are high-pressured inside your head, this will be evident to the sick person, who is likely to think, *This person wants to move along and doesn't want to be bothered with me.* What a conversation stopper!

How does Randy remain upbeat when dealing with other people who just don't get it?

"It's a mistake to ever expect it to be easy," he says. "We so desperately want it to be easy. The first line in Scott Peck's book *The Road Less Traveled* is, 'Life is difficult.' Once you grasp that, then it is supposed to be easier. But I find that it is still difficult, even after you grasp that it is difficult. We live in an ever-expanding horizon of difficulties. And with that we learn God's grace in all the ways that we don't want to see God's grace, because what we want is for Susan to be healed, and we tend to be blind to all the ways in which God's grace comes to us, even though Susan is not completely healed."

Randy is a highly spiritual man. For him the Bible is a rich resource. He used to be puzzled over why there were two opposite proverbs side by side. Proverbs 26:4 says, "Do not answer a fool according to his folly." The very next proverb says the opposite, "Answer a fool according to his folly."

"I finally realized," says Randy, "that perhaps it means that no matter how you deal with a fool, you lose. You are darned if you do and darned if you don't. Whether you talk to them or not, they still don't get it.

"Other people don't realize the magnitude of Susan's disability. They tend to view her deficits as showing either that she doesn't care or that she has character flaws. It feels as if you can't win with these people. They are not bad people. They simply live in a different world and suffer from a failure of imagination such that they cannot appreciate what life is like for us. They think they are putting themselves in our shoes, yet they have no idea what it would feel like to stand in our shoes. They actually believe they are being helpful when they say, 'Buck up!' They have no idea how devastating such comments can be. Someone should tell them, 'You are tromping like elephants on ground where angels fear to tread!'

"Jesus faced constant misunderstanding, yet he managed to love people anyway," Randy continues. "When you are in the midst of people who don't understand, sometimes you take a step back and try to accommodate the other person's weakness. That is hard when their weakness is hurting you, just because the other person is stubborn.

"Peter said to Jesus, 'Lord, to whom shall we go?' [John 6:68]. And we find the same thing. When people have once again failed us, when the church body has once again failed us, where else can we turn but to the Lord? This is the process of sanctification. That kind of self-discipline doesn't come easy. People give you lots of opportunities to have a less than godly response to them.

"With so many people around us who don't understand or worse, who set about to sabotage our efforts to survive, we had to become selective about who we let in, to be around us. The ones who aren't sympathetic tend to simply disappear from our life anyway.

"You have to discipline your thoughts not to go in the direction of being fed up with people," Randy says. "That is easy for me because I am a born optimist, a glass-half-full kind of person. I try to find something positive in the other person. But you eventually reach a certain resignation, recognizing that most people simply aren't going to understand."

Strategy Twenty: Use Your Suffering to Help Others

One way to deal with people who don't understand your suffering is to use your suffering to help others, which is the last strategy in our list of twenty. I will tell you four stories to illustrate it.

Sherri Connell's Writing

Sherri Connell of Parker, Colorado, has several debilitating illnesses including multiple sclerosis and advanced Lyme disease. Since there is no visible evidence of her problems, people often think she is wimpy and lazy. Her healthy friends have rejected her.

When Sherri's avalanche of disasters struck in her late twenties, she felt she had lost everything. Previously she had been an ambitious model, actress, playwright, and businesswoman. Then she had to watch in horror as those careers went down the drain. Her ability to have children was lost as was her energy and comfort in her body. Being rejected by her friends simply added insult to injury.

"One day my husband, Wayne, came to me with an idea," Sherri says. "From the time I was first diagnosed with multiple sclerosis, I started writing in my journal here and there, regarding living with chronic illness. Wayne suggested that we put some of my thoughts on the Internet. At first, I thought he was nuts! 'Who would want to see it?' I asked. After all, the World Wide Web is huge and why would anyone care what a disabled woman had to say?"

Despite Sherri's reservations, Wayne helped her create the site: The Invisible Disabilities Advocate at www.InvisibleDisabilities.org. It was an instant success, with tens of thousands of visitors per month. Many people suffering from similar maladies logged on and found solace in Sherri's writings. Wayne put some of her thoughts together into a booklet, "Have a Little Faith!"[5] In this way Sherri found a purpose and meaning that made sense out of her suffering. She was able to distill her experience and offer it online as a medicine to help others.

"My vision was narrow," Sherri admits, "but God took this little fish and loaf of bread and multiplied it beyond belief! I never could have imagined that from my home, sprawled across my chair, with messy clothes and dirty hair, my thoughts could reach out to thousands of hurting people! The Lord is using me in a much mightier, more vital way than being on Broadway, in a magazine, or on some commercial ever could have done!"

What does Sherri's website say that others find so helpful? Here's a sample:

> When a person loses their job or is forced to give up their career due to illness, people often treat them like they are choosing to do so. . . . Most people do not "give in" to illness. In fact, it is ingrained in our nature to fight to survive as hard and as long as humanly possible. . . . Creating limitations for oneself is one of the hardest things a person can do. It goes against everything we are and everything we ever hoped to be. No one wants to be sick and no one ever chooses to give up those things in life which bring such joy.
>
> What can sometimes be even harder to bear than the illness itself is feeling alone in the daily struggle and mourning of lifelong dreams. As pieces of oneself die off bit by bit, isolation consumes [sick people] when others refuse to affirm their pain. By repeatedly trying to "cheer them up" and make them see the "bright side," you are not validating their pain, but instead saying, "I don't want to hear the truth" or "your losses don't matter."[6]

Her advice to healthy people is: "You will never grasp what it is like to watch your lifetime dreams come crashing down forever. So stop using the excuse that you do not have understanding and start focusing on whether or not you have compassion!"[7]

Sherri discovered another reason that people were rejecting her. Some Christians assumed that a sick Christian who was not healed after praying for healing must be under God's judgment because of sin or insufficient faith. As if multiple sclerosis weren't enough, Sherri has to suffer the animosity of some Christians who, instead of being compassionate, are judgmental and hostile. When Christians pray for healing, they must realize that God answers the majority of such prayers with a no. Christians sometimes refuse to accept God's answer and blame the sick person for remaining sick.

This negative attitude toward sick people is found in the Bible! It is the attitude of Job's friend Eliphaz the Temanite and his sidekicks Bildad and Zophar. These so-called friends offer Job the same arguments that many Christians use today: that his persistent illness proves that Job must have offended God. What is God's attitude toward these judgmental advisors? "I am angry with you and your two friends," the Lord says to Eliphaz, "because you have not spoken of me what is right, as my servant Job has" (Job 42:7).

At the risk of being redundant, let me say that Sherri finds two reasons that healthy people are contemptuous toward her, a person with a chronic illness:

1. Sherri's disability is invisible.
2. Bad theology concerning healing leads to rejection by fellow Christians.

Because of the second issue, Sherri and Wayne launched a second website: Where Is God? (www.WhereIsGod.net). On this site Sherri writes about her belief that God could heal her, but when she has prayed for that, God's answer is no. God has other plans, Sherri says.

"I learned that true faith means believing that God knows best, even when he tells us no." Sherri cites the proverb that says, "Trust in the LORD with all your heart and lean not on your own understanding" (Prov. 3:5).

"When you pray for me," Sherri writes, "please do not just pray for healing; also pray for perseverance, joy, and peace. We need God's strength to endure the constant storm, until God decides to remove our pain."[8]

Sherri and I correspond. When she learned I was a psychiatrist, she wrote, "Please pray for me. I am a prisoner of my own broken body. My doc wants to put me on Serzone, but I am afraid it will increase my already unbearable dizziness, fatigue, exhaustion, and brain dysfunction. I feel like if I tell him no, he will label me as 'uncooperative' or 'malingering.' I tried many drugs and the side effects were not worth it. None made me feel better . . . just worse." Subsequently Sherri did try Serzone, but the side effects were intolerable, as she feared.

Before her illness Sherri was ambitious, goal-oriented, and a workaholic. Since her illness she writes, "I continue to mourn my business and theatre ministry. Not only that, it also grieves me to miss out on social activities, singing, and having children. I even mourn the loss of being able to do things that everyone else resents and complains about like cleaning, cooking, shopping, and running errands! Not an hour goes by that I don't come up against things I can no longer do. I will be honest: It is so very difficult to see everyone around me striving to 'do it all,' when I am to the point that I would be happy with just 'some of it.'"[9]

What excites Wayne and Sherri today is that they receive countless emails and letters from people living with chronic conditions, as well as spouses, siblings, physicians, and other authors, saying that these websites have changed their lives! The websites have yielded a plentiful harvest.

Janine Jacobsen's Counseling

Janine Jacobsen of Aurora, Colorado, has had Crohn's disease since childhood. After eighteen operations she has only two feet of small intestine left, which is not enough to sustain life. She needs additional nutrition, which she gets through a tube into a vein in her shoulder. Her medical problems are more severe than most people with Crohn's, because of "short bowel syndrome," which simply means that she has so little bowel left. She has other complications from decades of treatment—osteoporosis, osteoarthritis, cataracts, fatty liver, and kidney problems.

At age sixty-three Janine prays that the Lord will grant her another ten years of life. "If the Lord gave me twenty years, I'd take it," she says, "but I have to be realistic. I could only live ten years by the Lord's mercy. I could die because my veins give out so that I can no longer receive tube feeding, or if my health insurance gives out and no longer covers the 1,300 dollars a week that my medicines cost. If the insurance stops paying for TPN [tube feeding] when I turn sixty-five, I'll be dead within three weeks. The day when the Lord wants me, that's the day I will die. I don't know if I can bargain with him.

"I haven't had a lovely life," she says, "but I'm still alive and kicking. You have to have a good sense of humor when you have this kind of problem for so many years."

Several things have sustained Janine, in addition to her sense of humor (strategy six). She has a supportive husband and a network of friends (strategy one). Seven years ago, when she miraculously survived an infection, some born-again Christians (Margo and Hal Irwin) witnessed to her, and Janine found Jesus, who has become the centerpiece of her life, a source of joy.

What I want to focus on here is how Janine has been sustained by volunteering to help other women adapt to having a colostomy or ileostomy. A colostomy or ileostomy is an opening in the skin to which the colon or ileum is attached, so that body wastes, which can no longer pass through the anus, go into a plastic bag attached to the person's abdominal skin. Understandably, an ostomy stirs up emotional and psychological issues. Janine helps other women make the transition.

She says, "My normal colon and rectal functions are no longer present. The stoma has no shutoff valve. Digestive contents pass out of my body through the stoma and are collected in a drainage bag, which I wear at all times. Learning to live with an ostomy may seem like a big thing, especially since it often leaks at the beginning until you get to know how to use the thing. But it is easier to get used to than you would imagine. My husband, Oddy, has been incredibly supportive and made me feel sexy and wanted. He is fond of saying, 'It is only a mechanical problem, so don't worry. Life is good and I love you.'"

The United Ostomy Association refers women to Janine who need to adjust to an ostomy. They try to match Janine with women of about the same age who have had a similar surgical procedure. She sees people from mid-forties to age seventy who are trying to get used to the idea of having a pouch. Women counsel women, and men talk to men. Janine says, "If you have an ostomy, then having the Ostomy Association in your life is a must."

Janine tries to see the newcomer at least two or three times in the person's home. She talks with family, friends, and anyone who is available. Her basic message is that an ostomy (wearing a pouch) is not a disaster, and in fact, it is a blessing! She bursts with enthusiasm. "Life is good. With a pouch you can live again. You no longer have the accidents and pain that were caused by the disease prior to getting an ostomy.

"Chronic pain is debilitating," she says. "Once you have the pouch, the pain is gone and you get your life back. Then it is important for your family and friends to begin to treat you again the way they used to treat you before you were subdued and debilitated by pain. It really is a joy to be alive, once you get rid of the pain."

When Janine first had an ostomy, there was no one to talk to. She didn't know anyone who had such a thing. It was appalling, so humiliating that she felt that she couldn't go on living. If a veteran had counseled her at the time of her first ostomy, the transition would have been easier.

Her first ostomy was temporary. When Janine had her second one, a woman named Timi Reves visited her in the hospital, which was enormously helpful. Timi's message was that Janine need not live in fear.

Now when Janine counsels women, her message is similar: things aren't as bad as they expect. Their fears are unfounded. There is no need to become housebound; they just need to know at all times where the nearest bathroom is. If Janine is in a crowded restaurant and there is a long line at the ladies' room, she goes to the woman at the head of the line and says, "Look, I have a pouch, so do you mind if I cut in?"

"The bottom line is that you need to have self-confidence, a sense of security in yourself," Janine says. "No one needs to know you wear a pouch unless you are like me and have a big mouth. I tell everyone."

What about sex? Janine counsels women based on her own experience. She wears something sexy to make love with her husband, so he doesn't ever see the pouch and there is only one part of her body he shouldn't touch. "If you had a good sex life before and your husband loves you, then nothing should change after you get the pouch," Janine says.

"Women get depressed," she continues. "But there is no need to. You can adjust. Life is just a little different. Your requirements are slightly different than they used to be. Take me for example. The ostomy does not prevent me from going swimming each day, boating, hiking, fishing, snowmobiling, traveling to Europe, taking cruises, cooking, painting in oils and watercolors, gardening, wearing blue jeans, or dressing up elegantly in tight outfits. My pouch is no obstacle to having an active life."

I asked Janine a stupid question. "Does helping other women with their ostomy help you live with your illness?" The reason it was stupid is that Janine doesn't volunteer in order to help herself. Yes, she feels good when she can help someone. Yes, she prays for and with the women she counsels. Yes, counseling other women allows her to use her own suffering to benefit others. But no, Janine does not do this volunteer work because it makes her feel better. She has never had such a thought. She simply helps others because it is the natural thing to do.

Janine admits, "Helping other women adapt to their ostomies is very rewarding. I enjoy visiting people. Through those visits I have made several friends."

Janine named her ostomy Charlie. Such a name allows her to keep her sense of humor and to recognize that she, not Charlie, is in charge. Every morning she says, "Charlie, now we are going to behave ourselves today, aren't we!" Usually, if Janine watches what she eats, she and Charlie get along pretty well. She encourages other women to give their ostomy a name so they can establish a collaborative relationship with it.

"You have to overcome fear," Janine says, "because life is so precious that you cannot waste it. When you get used to a pouch, the fears evaporate and the pain vanishes as if it had never existed. You forget that you have an invisible illness. Life is delicious!"

Janine has other things to teach about how to enjoy life despite Crohn's disease. She finds that forgiving her enemies helps. Her father beat her mother and Janine when she was a child, she explains. As an adult she discovered that hatred was bad for her health. Her life improved when she forgave her father, thereby getting rid of the hatred that was gnawing at her from the inside.

"I love this passage from the New Testament," Janine says. "We . . . rejoice in our sufferings, because we know that suffering produces perseverance; perseverance, character; and character, hope" (Rom. 5:3–4).

Pat Mierop, a Prayer Warrior

"God is frugal," Pat says. "He wastes nothing, and he doesn't want us to waste our pain." Sitting at home alone, blind from diabetes, Pat tells me that her illnesses are blessings since her suffering has prepared her to comfort younger women who turn to her for help in her ministry as a prayer warrior.

A malignant tumor laid waste Pat's left eye seven years before bleeding inside her right eye plunged her into darkness in less than a half hour. "The first evening I went to bed blind," Pat said, "a friend who was staying with me that night came into the bedroom and turned out the light. I didn't know it had been on!

"God doesn't make mistakes," Pat continues. "My blindness taught me how God can provide. Immediately, people came from our church to take care of me. I taught them how to test my blood sugar and adjust the amount of insulin. I never knew we had so many nurses in our church. God may have hemmed me in, but he has not put me on the shelf. He has a different plan for me.

"A Christian nurse asked me whether I was angry at God for afflicting me," she says. "That isn't a Christian way to think. We need to remember who God is and trust that he's working for the best, even when we can't see yet how things fit together. We should wait on God. For me insulin is a blessing. Without it I couldn't live. And my blindness brought people into my house all day long, accelerating my ministry of prayer with younger women whose pain I would not be able to comprehend if I had no hardships."

Pat cites Mary Gardiner Brainard's "Not Knowing" poem:

I'd rather walk in the dark with God than to walk alone in the light.
I'd rather walk with Him by faith than to walk alone by sight.

After Pat prayed for the ability to read the Bible again, the blood inside one of her eyes slowly cleared. "Over a period of many months, I went from blackness to heavy shadows and light," she said, "to the return of splotches of color, to vague shapes and indistinct faces, to finally being able to read with very bright light. God has graciously enabled me to read again. That's what I asked for."

She is just barely able to read. She cannot drive. She tells me that it takes humility to ask God to meet her practical needs, but it takes even more humility to ask family and friends.

Sherri's, Janine's, and Pat's stories illustrate one of the most powerful strategies of sick people: using their suffering to help others. Isaiah wrote about the suffering servant (52:13–53:12)—the wounded healer. Jesus picked up the theme (Matt. 20:26–28; Mark 10:43–45; John 13:2–17). He also said, "It is more blessed to give than to receive" (Acts 20:35). Now many sick people minister to others as suffering servants and are blessed.

Father John Cockayne, Catholic Priest

After one of my public talks about this book, a woman in the audience went home and talked to her priest, Father John Cockayne of St. Thomas Catholic Church in Thomaston, Connecticut. Out of the blue he phoned me, bursting with enthusiasm. "A double thumbs up!" he said on my answering machine, "my deepest shalom." His voice was thready, wobbly, and difficult to understand. He said he suffered from chronic illnesses and invited me to contact him to see if there was any way that he could help me with this project.

When I returned his phone call, I found John to be nearly euphoric about the opportunity to talk with me. He had already been praying for the success of this book.

John told me he was fifty-one years old, and implied that he had a hundred-and-two-year-old body, though he exhibited the spirit of a twenty-one-year-old. He was born with cerebral palsy, which was why he had a slight speech impediment despite thousands of hours of speech therapy. As he aged, he was afflicted with worsening arthritis, and his gait was spastic and irregular. Recently he had become diabetic, which meant that he was more vulnerable to infection—bronchitis, pneumonia, and other infections—from which he had suffered throughout his life.

After college in Seneca Falls, New York, John pursued a master of public administration degree. He spent seven years working with people with disabilities. When he was twenty-seven, he had a bout with the flu and was stuck at home, watching lots of TV. Pope John Paul II was visiting Boston and New York at the time, and some of his speeches were televised. John was impressed, especially by his talk at Yankee Stadium. As a result, John's prayer life became more intense. Every day he took the Eucharist at his church. Within a year he phoned the archdiocese saying he wanted to become a priest. Then he went to seminary for four years and was ordained at age thirty-two.

Because he has been sick his entire life, John takes illness for granted. There is none of that sense of disappointment that I find with someone who was previously healthy and now has to adjust to sickness and disability. Through his prayer life, John manages to keep going. When I interviewed him, he was recovering from his latest bout of pneumonia.

He says, "I simply do the best that I can." In other words, John accepts the limitations that the Lord has imposed on his life. "I am frustrated at times," he says, "because the spirit wants to do everything, but the body is weak." His sense of humor and love of his vocation help him through the hard times.

"I am interested in spirituality and suffering," John says. "Our religion is about the cross, passion, and death. It is also about resurrection and hope. This gives me a sense of direction. Consider the Stations of the Cross. We don't know for sure that Christ fell three times on his way to Calvary, but the Stations of the Cross portray him falling three times. Each time it was more difficult for him to get back on his feet, but he got up three times. This means that it is all right to fall, to succumb to anguish and pain. Repeatedly we need to struggle to our feet again, to continue our journey. If we try our best to struggle and cope, God will honor our efforts.

"When I visit the homebound," John continues, "I tell them that it is not always important to do things physically to serve God. People who are homebound can serve God through prayer. Even suffering can be a form of prayer. It is a form of ministry just to lift up your suffering and offer it to God."

"Do you mean that God can use someone's suffering to help others?" I ask. "Are you saying that if someone who is isolated at home humbly offers her or his pain and anxiety up to God, that can be used by God to help a different person whom you don't know and have never met?"

"One would hope so," John replies. "It is a mystery. We won't know for sure about these things until we meet God face-to-face. Maybe when we do meet him, we will be so happy that we won't even care about how he used our former suffering. Meanwhile on this earth we deal with human emotions, like pain and anxiety. Intellectually it is hard to know what spiritual benefit God derives from us lifting up our suffering, but there is some definite benefit.

"This is why the Christian community is so important," John continues. "We can use the patient suffering of the saints as examples to inspire us and help us carry on. I am not just referring to the canonized saints. Ordinary Christians bear witness by struggling to carry on as best they can.

"Everyone would prefer a physical healing, but God heals in many different ways, not just physically. There are many ways of growing from suffering and pain. You can be healed spiritually. You can grow to understand that whereas this dimension of your life may be limited, maybe there are other dimensions that will flower with new possibilities.

"My disability is a gift," John says. "It gives me greater sensitivity and awareness of the needs of others. I always say that if you strike out the letter *D* from the word *disabled*, you get the words *is able*.

"Everyone is created in the image and likeness of God. We use our gifts and our limitations to try to make a difference. Sometimes our limitations *are* gifts. They create a tension or balance between the spirit and the body."

"What ongoing problems do you have?" I ask.

"My problem is that I am better at reading other people's needs than I am at paying attention to my own," John says. "I tell others that they need to allow the space and time to heal. Then I forget that advice when it comes to me. As I grow older, I am beginning to acquire wisdom about the need to take care of myself also, so as to be more effective as a person."

After John had worked nineteen years as assistant priest in different churches, the Diocese of Hartford wanted to promote him in a way that would support him. Given his illnesses, they knew they couldn't make him the solo priest at a church. He needed backup because of his unpredictable sick time. So they arranged for Father Maynard Kearns at St. Thomas to step down from being the administrative priest to become the assistant, and they promoted John from being assistant to the top position. St. Thomas is a church of sixteen hundred people. This meant that John had to face problems he'd never dealt with previously, such as responsibility for a huge budget, a budget deficit, the task of laying off some staff, and the need to plan a capital fund drive to renovate the aging church building.

As John began to shoulder these mind-boggling responsibilities, he had a bout of bronchitis, a urinary tract infection, worsening neck pain, and for the first time ever he got depressed and began having panic attacks. Father Kearns took over the helm and John went on extended sick leave, visiting his parents in Florida to recover. He was placed on Effexor and entered psychotherapy with a psychologist. The bronchitis went away, the depression subsided, and John began to see light at the end of the tunnel.

The archdiocese is telling him to take as much time as he needs to get his strength back. As of today John is undecided whether to return immediately to being the administrative priest at St. Thomas or whether to take a six-month sabbatical to study and regroup. During his nineteen years in the priesthood, John has never taken any vacation time at all.

As we sat together at lunch, John mused about his recent illness. "I think I just said one time too many, if you excuse my language, 'Damn the torpedoes, full speed ahead!'" John said, explaining why he got depressed. "The Lord said to me, 'You are going to take the time and space to regroup until you are feeling better and reach a better level of wholeness.'

"Chronic illness is like a roller coaster," John says. "There is a grieving process. Sometimes you can accept it. Sometimes you are upset with God. That is healthy. You have to try to pick up the pieces and continue in the great virtues of faith, hope, and love. You can't candy coat chronic illness.

"I try to help people make sense of their chronic pain and illness. The main thing is not to become discouraged, to encourage optimism, to be hope filled. I think of the song, 'I Never Promised You a Rose Garden.' Even roses get diseases and Japanese beetles. You have to fertilize roses and water them properly. That is what life is all about—making the most of it, using the ups, downs, and challenges to bring a better quality of life to others. My own strength and optimism are coming back now.

"When I celebrate the Sacraments," John goes on, "such as anointing the sick, I believe that prayer and laying on of hands might bring the ability to cope with a situation. I share my pilgrimage with people. I don't know if this helps them. But I hope it does."

At the end of our lunch John holds both my hands and prays. As we hold hands, I notice that John's elbows are oscillating and his wrists and hands are wiggling from cerebral palsy.

"May the Lord bless you and keep you," John says. "May his face shine upon you and be gracious to you. May he hold you and your family close to his heart and in the palm of his hands. May the Holy Spirit continue to empower you. And may the Lord use this book to help many people."

EPILOGUE

A year after I interviewed John, I phoned him, and we scheduled another meeting over lunch. He had a lot to tell me. He has resigned as administrative priest at St. Thomas church. I think that was a good idea, since the job description didn't seem to fit him in my view. He says he's feeling better but is still on a health sabbatical. Recently he celebrated mass on TV. The Archbishop remains very supportive of John, even when John says he wants to leave the parish ministry and develop a career of offering spiritual enrichment to people with disabilities and chronic illnesses. John has been spending time studying in the libraries of Yale Divinity School and Hartford Seminary. He has been fascinated with the idea for my book since he first heard about it and is reading about the impact of the epidemic of chronic illness on healthcare finances.

10

Two Themes
and Two Conclusions

Two Themes

The Centers for Disease Control (CDC) define chronic conditions as those that "are prolonged, do not resolve spontaneously, and are rarely cured completely."[1] This book makes two proposals. I propose that there is an increasing epidemic in the number of people living with chronic illnesses, which means that we need to learn how to live with these diseases. The other proposal is that by listening to people who have successfully adapted to such illnesses, we can learn twenty strategies for doing the same.

Theme One: Being Sick Well

Having a chronic disease is like having a career. You can do poorly or well at it.

The stories of people in this book have focused on a few people whom my friends referred to me because they managed somehow to live well, not in the sense that their incurable illness was cured

231

but in the sense of the spiritual virtues they developed. I interviewed these people seeking to learn how they adjusted to their illnesses. There was no set list of questions that I asked. I had no preconceived ideas. By telling their stories, I hope that I have allowed the reader to look through the eyes of my interviewees and feel what it would be like to walk in their shoes.

Sherri Connell, in chapter 9, asked me to write a preface for her book *But You Look So Good*. Here is part of what I wrote: "Sometimes a person's character is not evident until thrown into the furnace of affliction. Like John Wayne's tough determination isn't evident in a movie until he is out-gunned ten to one. That is part of what makes Sherri Connell's story so compelling. Against all odds she emerges as a determined woman of real grit, capable of taking on the meanest that life has to throw at her, and still surfacing with heroic courage after getting hit by a tsunami."[2]

The sick people I interviewed live interesting and inspiring lives. They demonstrate the nobility of the human spirit on the medical battlefield. Taking them as my teachers, I learned twenty strategies they employed to achieve the success they did.

There are other strategies that could be included, such as listening to music, having a pet, keeping a journal, and adhering to your diet. I didn't make a list of strategies and then go out to find people to illustrate them. My approach was the opposite. I interviewed anyone referred to me and learned the strategies from them. Only a third of the people I interviewed are found in this book. Among the many case histories I wrote, I chose to use those that were colorful and memorable, as well as ones that taught an important lesson that might be useful to the reader.

One example of how someone with a chronic illness might benefit from studying this book is me. For the past fifty years I have suffered from bouts of major depression. This disease is subtle in the way it infiltrates my brain. It does not always have obvious symptoms. Rather it insidiously and drearily colors my perception of the world, like the paintings from Picasso's blue period. This makes it easy for me to see people as more hostile than they are, and current events as more alarming than they are. Like Richard Geiger in chapter 7, I have suffered from a mysterious distortion in my ability to see reality, biasing me in a pessimistic direction. As a result, whenever I have a pessimistic thought, it triggers a mistrust of my own thinking. Antidepressant medicines, psychotherapy, and exercise have helped but have not rid me of my tendency toward dejection.

More than anything else, the people I interviewed for this book have helped me. The twenty strategies, when applied to my life, have lifted me out of depression. This book has been for me my own version of Complementary and Alternative Medicine.

Years ago I married Maureen, who is delightful. With her I have another child, Matthew, who is eleven years old. These two have buoyed my spirits. Felicity, my daughter with Pat, is thriving and happy at age thirty-two. Felicity got her Ph.D. in biostatistics and just got married to Patrick Enders, a wonderful physician with whom Pat would have been delighted.

Living with a chronic illness is not drastically different from living with unemployment, a bad boss, a bad marriage, poverty, imprisonment, an unresolved lawsuit, amidst a civil war, or other trials and tribulations. And the strategies presented in this book could benefit those struggling with other forms of affliction.

Chronic illness can be viewed as a metaphor for life itself. For example, a nurse who works with me says that I should write another book with the subtitle, "Joyful Living despite Chronic Parenting." Two of her grown children recently moved back home.

The idea that some people live acceptable lives despite chronic illness is only one of the themes of this book. The second theme concerns the increasing epidemic of chronic illnesses, which makes the first theme more important.

Theme Two: The Epidemic

In the introduction and chapter 4 I set forth the evidence that there is an epidemic of chronic illness. The data indicate that 45 percent of the population has at least one chronic condition, and that percentage is increasing.

One of the mysteries this book has addressed is how such a massive epidemic, which is the most glaring and conspicuous thing going on in health today, could be so little recognized and discussed so infrequently. Part of the reason for the invisibility of this epidemic is that when we think of chronic illness, our minds play a trick on us. We tend to think of catastrophic illness. The dramatic and tragic cases stick in our minds. Most of the popular books on the subject mistakenly focus on devastating diseases, as if those were typical. In reality only a minority of people with chronic conditions have disastrous lives. The term *chronic illness* means something different to laypeople than it does to medical professionals, who know that it means long-term but not necessarily catastrophic. The most common chronic condition is high blood pressure, which usually causes no symptoms at all. That's why the high numbers of chronic sufferers are difficult to recognize, because people who appear to be healthy have high blood pressure, asthma, arthritis, and a myriad of other common problems.

I do not mean to make chronic illness sound trivial. This book is loaded with case histories of people with devastating illnesses. But it is important to see the big picture, and catastrophic illness is not typical. More typical is your neighbor who looks healthy, works full time, takes sick time, and never talks to you about the pills and inhalers she uses every day to keep the beast under control.

My friend Dr. Andrew Greenhill from Pittsburgh, Pennsylvania, provides an illustration that helps explain why this epidemic is invisible. At age fifty-seven Andy is a veteran of the war with chronic illness. By rearranging his life, he has kept his diseases under control and has lived a full and rewarding life.

When he was twenty-seven, during his pediatric internship, Andy developed ulcerative colitis. For decades after that he took an orange pill called sulfasalazine. "I took so much of that stuff that I used to joke with Ann, saying that my bones were orange," he says. The onset of ulcerative colitis seemed to confirm Andy's lifelong expectation that he would die at an early age. Although he didn't die, it confirmed his idea that he was a vulnerable person.

"The disease regulated my life," Andy told me. He described his need to always know where the nearest toilet was located and his difficulty jogging or traveling if he didn't have that information. After thirty years with ulcerative colitis, it subsided. "If you don't have a severe case and if you don't get cancer," he said, "ulcerative colitis eventually burns itself out."

Despite this disease, Andy's life flourished. He was happily married to one of the most delightful women I've ever met, Ann Hirsh. During his pediatric residency at Case Western Reserve Medical School, they lived in the other half of the duplex house that Pat and I lived in when I was in medical school. Our daughter, Felicity, age two, used to call them "AnnNAndy" as if they shared one name. After Cleveland, Andy took specialized fellowships, first in pediatric nephrology, then in allergy. He worked as an allergist for decades in Davis, California, where they raised their two children, Leah and David. Despite his bowel problems, Andy always jogged thirty to thirty-five miles a week.

He describes himself as a cultural Jew. He says he is an atheist who thinks of himself as a good person because he embraces the values of Judaism. "I am neither spiritual nor ritualistic," he says. "I don't believe there is a God who oversees my life. So I never question why I developed these diseases. It's just the cards I was dealt, based on genetics and environmental factors." When Andy and Ann attended Congregation Bet Haverim in Davis, their primary motivation was to provide religious education for their children.

At age forty-eight Andy developed angina. It was an eerie, chilly sensation that would creep up his neck into his jaw when he was jogging the first mile. "I went in for a cardiac cath," he said. "They found a blockage in many arteries, especially the left main coronary artery, which is called the 'widow-maker,' because if it closes, your entire left ventricle has no blood supply. I had six-vessel bypass surgery." Aware that he could die if this invisible disease progressed, Andy shaped his life around the need to control the risk factors for hardening of the arteries.

"Ann says I always do things in extremes," Andy says. "Like, if I make a salad, I throw in every kind of vegetable I can find. So I took an extreme approach to cardiac rehab. Within a week of the surgery I was out walking. The next week I was jogging a little, but it hurt to breathe. I was gasping for air. By six weeks I was running six miles a day. I changed my diet, following the books of Dean Ornish. The cardiologists said to do things in moderation, taking less than 30 percent of calories in fat. But I never ate that much fat to begin with. I went to the extreme and reduced my fat intake to less than ten grams a day. I try to control everything I can. That is my compensating mechanism. It's how I cope."

Maureen and I had Ann and Andy over for dinner. Andy ate no meat. He nibbled on some bread, salad, and rice. He was extremely thin, looking undernourished, like someone with anorexia. The experts say you are healthier if you are under- rather than overnourished. I've always struggled with the opposite problem—overnourished. I wish I had Andy's self-discipline.

He still runs a seven-minute mile for at least four miles a day, five or more days a week. My walking half an hour a day seems paltry and slovenly knowing that in the same time Andy will have run four miles, during the first mile of which he may have angina.

"In addition to exercise and diet," Andy says, "Ornish tells his readers to reduce the amount of stress in their lives. I tried meditation, but I never could achieve that inward focus and concentration. So I reduced my medical practice from sixty hours a week to thirty-five. I eliminated all administrative responsibilities for our group practice. Eventually I retired from Davis so that we could move to Pittsburgh to live three blocks from our daughter, Leah, who is doing an ophthalmology residency. Her husband, Andrew, is doing an internal medicine residency. They no longer had the time to travel to see us in California. Our children are our priority in life. We moved to live near them, to try to help make their lives easier. Then I was offered a job as an allergist at one of the University of Pittsburgh hospitals. Now I work between one and one-and-a-half days a week. That's ideal for me."

Our conversation over the dinner table rambles over many topics.

"I have many degrees," Ann laughs. "I have a DD for being a doctor's daughter, and a DS for being a doctor's sister. Of course I have a DW for being a doctor's wife, a DM for being a doctor's mother, and a DML for being a doctor's mother-in-law." Her comment reminds me that Ann is the most family-oriented person I ever met. She has many other accomplishments, including a master's degree in speech pathology. She spent fifteen years running a respite program for developmentally disabled children in Davis.

If you met Dr. Andy Greenhill, you would never guess that his life has been shaped around his two illnesses, unless he told you. His life demonstrates why chronic illness is such an invisible problem. You go to see your allergist. You rely on him. It never crosses your mind that he has been living with two major-league diseases for decades. He looks completely healthy!

Two Conclusions

There are two conclusions that can be derived from the twenty strategies that form the backbone of this book. The first is that the burden imposed by a disease can sometimes be modified. The second is that the basic music of life is joyful. These two conclusions are my way of boiling the twenty strategies down to their essence.

Burdens Can Become Lighter

Figure 10 shows two different theories about how an illness is related to the burden that the illness imposes. I use the word *burden* to mean the extent to which an illness is emotionally difficult to bear, a source of misery, distress, and unhappiness. The burden of an illness is the extent to which it weighs down the human spirit, crushes you, and grinds you down. Theory A at the top of the illustration shows a direct relationship between the illness and the burden. This is the view that most people have when they first get sick. Because they are sick, they are burdened (or disabled) to some extent, and they believe that nothing can be done about it until the sickness is cured.

Theory A is poisonous if you have a chronic illness. It leads to a stalemate and feelings of powerlessness, hopelessness, and resignation. If the illness is not cured and may not be curable, you are left with the sense that there is nothing to do but suffer.

Fortunately theory A is wrong! The bottom half of figure 10 illustrates theory B, which is the viewpoint that I hold. It shows that illness leads to burden, but a multitude of other factors, including strategies in this book, can modify and lighten the burden.

Jesus implies that a burden can be either heavy or light. He says, "Come to me, all you who are weary and burdened, and I will give you rest. Take my yoke upon you and learn from me, for I am gentle and humble in heart, and you will find rest for your souls. For my yoke is easy and my burden is light" (Matt. 11:28–30). When someone is weary from carrying a heavy load and they are spiritually renewed, their load can seem light. That's what this book is all about.

Figure 10

Two Theories of the Burden of Illness

Theory A

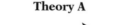

Illness ━━━━━━━━━▶ Burden of Illness

Theory B

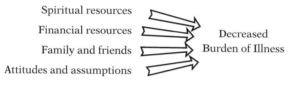

Spiritual resources

Financial resources ━━━▶ Decreased

Family and friends ━━━▶ Burden of Illness

Attitudes and assumptions

GARY POVIRK

A friend of mine, Gary Povirk, suffers from fibromyalgia. I mention him because he demonstrates that the burden of pain is modifiable. When I first met Gary, he was doing metallurgy research on the faculty of Yale University. He was so fatigued by his pain that it was one of the defining issues of his life. His doctors had no way to relieve his discomfort.

Like many people with fibromyalgia, Gary surfed the net, looking for some solution. A fellow fibromyalgia sufferer advised him to routinize his life: Always get up at the same time, eat at the same time every day, and so on. Gary gave it a try. He began waking up at the same time every morning and following the same schedule of meals. Also he renegotiated his relationship with his wife, Lisa, with whom he had a rather rocky marriage. He left Yale to work for a military contractor who offered more financial rewards with a less demanding work schedule. In addition, Gary slowly increased his daily physical exercise.

These changes did not occur overnight, nor were they easy. There was a lot of trial and error. When he first started exercising, he hurt his hip, then his calf muscles and tendons. For a while he had to stop. Then he discovered that taking a hot bath before exercise warmed up his muscles. He developed a series of seven exercises that he did, one each night of the week. Slowly, against all odds, he persisted and learned that he could start walking on a regular basis, then running!

Research on fibromyalgia shows that regular exercise is one of the few things that helps in the long run. This is difficult because people with fibromyalgia don't feel like exercising. When they begin exercising, they often experience a flare-up of their symptoms the next day. But a commitment to a discipline of exercise, starting gently and ever so slowly increasing over time, has been shown in research studies to yield positive results for that particular illness.

If a doctor had told Gary, "You need to exercise," that advice would have had little impact. He had to figure it out on his own. He designed a program that prevented his disease from getting worse and actually made it considerably less restricting.

When Gary began trying to regularize his sleeping schedule, he would get exhausted during the day. He learned to fight through that and avoid taking naps, so that he could sleep only at night according to plan. His guiding principle was to develop a consistent daily routine.

When Gary and I were together, we took a brisk ninety-minute walk. A year earlier such a walk would have left him depleted and exhausted for days. But this time I could barely keep up with him, and he felt great! He is now able to live a full life despite fibromyalgia, finding that the effects of the disease are not set in concrete, that there was something he could do to improve his condition.

The idea that the burden of illness can be modified is one of the two conclusions that can be derived from this book. How to accomplish that varies from person to person and from disease to disease. You may believe there is nothing you can do to change your situation. Gary Povirk gave up being longsuffering and learned how to master his disease. He did so by paying attention to and changing the things that added to the burden, from his unsatisfying marriage, his employment and career goals, to his daily schedule and exercise.

Making a distinction between a chronic condition and the burden caused by that condition is important because you may not be able to do much about your illness, but a careful analysis of the burden often reveals that it can be modified. Your lifestyle, attitude, social network, and the skill with which you manage your disease are more closely related to the burden than is the illness itself, as we learn from

Gary. Living with an illness can be experienced as a noble or ignoble task, humanizing or dehumanizing, causing you to feel on the one hand heroic and courageous or on the other hand diminished and worthless. Sometimes you oscillate between these emotions.

Sickness is like warfare. The battlefield is not simply a place where people are wounded, killed, terrified, or angry. It is also a place for unprecedented heroism. Some soldiers who receive the Purple Heart or the Congressional Medal of Honor had no idea that there was a heroic bone in their body. Until they found themselves on the firing line, they thought of themselves as cowards or simply ordinary. But the horror of a battlefield tests the stuff of which you are made, and some people are astonished to find courage in their guts.

We don't give the equivalent of a Purple Heart to those who are heroic with their chronic diseases. But we should! If we gave more recognition and public acclaim to the kind of people found in this book, that recognition would inspire other sick people and caregivers to say, "Doggone it. I don't need to be crushed and defeated by this disease!"

One key to happiness despite chronic illness is to recognize that crushing burden is not an inevitable part of illness. While writing this book I met many people who experience the weight of their cross as light. They are some of the most awesome and inspiring people that I have ever met.

PLACIDO MASTROIANNI

As I was finishing the writing of this book, I had another haircut with Placido Mastroianni, my longtime barber. I have lots of hair and it grows fast, so Placido and I see one another often. For him the "burden" caused by his diseases is encompassed almost entirely in his lower boccie score. He tells me that he kept working at it, playing boccie three times every week. It was humiliating to have the ball catapult off in a different direction than he wanted because of the lack of coordination of his right arm caused by the stroke he suffered twelve years ago.

"Those guys don't care whether or not I had a stroke," he says. "They simply want to win. They say nasty things if I drag down the score."

Five years after his stroke Placido noticed his game was improving. Year in and year out he kept practicing, about fifteen hundred days of playing boccie since his stroke. Slowly Placido learned how to work around his deficit. He discovered that he lost control of the ball only if he bowled fast. His style had always been to bowl fast. But he taught himself to throw the boccie balls slower but with greater accuracy.

"My boccie score now is almost back 100 percent," he says, beaming, and even more animated than usual. "It's taken twelve years, Doc, but I'm almost back to my old skill level. Just yesterday I made a mistake, but I was able to recover. The other team had three balls close to the little ball, which in Italian we call it the *pallino*, which means 'little.' I thought I could get my boccie ball past the *pallino* and knock their ball away. But I had to throw very close to the *pallino*, and I missed and hit the *pallino* ball instead, so it rolled even closer to the other team's balls. So then it was a real tight spot! But I concentrated, bowled slowly, and made a very difficult shot, getting my ball between the *pallino* and the other team's boccie balls. So I recovered the mistake. And we won!"

That news made me happier than I've ever been leaving Placido's barbershop, and I always leave there happy.

Life Can Be Victorious

The second conclusion we can derive from this book is that the basic music of life is joyful. As Harold Koenig says, we live in a benevolent universe.[3] Thus it is possible to live a victorious instead of a defeated life.

Every morning I read the *New York Times*. The front-page news is usually grim. If I were to base my view of reality on that newspaper, or any news media, I would think that life is tragic, and human nature ugly. For me this is a big issue, because my father, who suffered from worse depression than me and was an atheist, taught me that life was a losing proposition. The front page of the *New York Times* usually confirmed his viewpoint.

An important change took place in my life my senior year of college, when Handel's *Messiah* led to my conversion from atheism to Christianity. At that point I shifted my view of reality. Instead of basing my perception on the *New York Times*, I based my view of life on the gospel. The word *gospel* means "good news." Changing my perception of life was one of the most basic steps in solving my problem of major depression. What the gospel and the Bible meant to me, personally, was that joy triumphed over defeat, resurrection over crucifixion, and eternal life over disease.

This book has presented case histories of people from the six major religions of the United States: Christianity, Judaism, Islam, Buddhism, Hinduism, and nonspecific spirituality. I tried to be fair and evenhanded in presenting the stories of people from each of these spiritual traditions. Since I am a Christian, it is the viewpoint I understand best.

The Bible gives me a foundation on which to stand, when I declare that we can find joy despite the *New York Times* and despite chronic illness. One of the basic themes of the Bible is that we should celebrate, rejoice, and give thanks for the abundant blessings God continues to shower on us. When I count how many times the Bible mentions the words *rejoice, joyful, glad, celebrate,* or *delight,* the answer is 748 times. The word *praise* occurs 403 times, bringing the total of these encouraging words to well over a thousand times.[4] As Pollyanna says, "If God took the trouble to tell us eight hundred times to be glad and rejoice, He must want us to do it."[5]

Do you think the basic energy of life is positive or negative? When we listen to the music of our lives, is the universe tuned to a major or a minor key? My ear hears a major key. Is the canvas of life painted with warm hues, such as yellow, orange, red, and light green? Or is it painted with cold hues, such as blues and grays? If you answer, "Mixed," then I ask you this question: Which hues are dominant? If you stand distant from your life and look at it, do you see a cheerful or a dreary picture? Now my picture of life is painted in warm hues.

In chapter 4 I presented the debate between other experts and me, concerning whether good news or bad news is dominant. On the one hand there are more and more people with chronic diseases, on the other hand there is a decreasing rate of disability among the elderly. In that chapter I was discussing the secular trends surrounding the worsening epidemic of chronic illness. I told you why several experts think I am too pessimistic.

But here I am discussing a different issue. Chapter 4 was about secular trends, whereas here I am talking about the sacred foundations for optimism. Thus you might say that I tend to be a secular pessimist (because we live in a fallen world) but a sacred optimist (because God will triumph in the end).

The growth of my optimism has been a major transformation for me, involving both my spiritual and psychological being. During my years with my wife Pat, as she deteriorated, I was sometimes depressed. But the depression never struck me as being compatible with the deepest harmonies of the universe. When I found joy, I felt more in sync with the wavelength of life itself (more in tune with God). Illness does not have the last word in my book. Joy is more abiding than tears.

I used to think that Shakespeare's tragedies were more compelling than his comedies. In Shakespeare's day the word *comedy* did not mean that something was funny. Rather, a comedy was a play that had a happy ending. Today I believe that Shakespeare saw his comedies as more compelling than his tragedies. Why? Because Shakespeare's play *A Midsummer Night's Dream* mocked *Romeo and Juliet*. *A Midsummer Night's Dream* contained a play within a play, called "Pyramus and Thisbe." It was a parody of *Romeo and Juliet*. Because Shakespeare's tragedies never mocked his comedies, we can see that comedy was more basic to Shakespeare's mind than tragedy.

Life, even life with a chronic disease, is more of a comedy than a tragedy, using the word *comedy* in the Shakespearean sense. By this I mean that there is a happy ending. To illustrate, let me tell you the last story of this book, a brief biography of Frank Fabiano.

FRANK FABIANO

Frank was a forty-five-year-old, obese man who worked as a unit clerk at my hospital. He was cheerful despite four massive heart attacks, bypass surgery, nineteen years of back pain, and five back surgeries. Frank knew his days were numbered, especially after he keeled over with a cardiac arrest in the middle of the nurse's station. Some nurses administered CPR. Frank was taken to the cardiac care unit and survived. An automatic defibrillator was implanted in his body, attached to his heart. Frank, laughing, told me that a couple of electrical jolts from the defibrillator was better than a cup of coffee for waking him up in the morning.

The hospital administration was reluctant to allow Frank to return to work. They considered it impolite for him to die in public. But

Frank insisted. He said he could not support his family on disability income, and besides, it was boring to sit around home waiting for the other shoe to drop. So before long, Frank was back on the job, resuming his role as a source of lightheartedness. When Frank came back to work, I felt that the sun started shining again.

Frank told me that he had nothing to worry about because he was in God's hands. If he died tomorrow, he would go to a better place, he said. Frank was Catholic. One day Frank didn't come to work. He had departed to that place where there is no disease (Rev. 22:1–3), where "there will be no more death or mourning or crying or pain" (Rev. 21:4).

THE SOURCE OF JOY

Most of the things reported in the *New York Times* are transient. They are part of a world that is passing away. Even chronic disease is fleeting. Life is brief. At times it may seem interminable, but then suddenly our children and grandchildren are grown up and the whole drama is over. The Bible says that we are like the grass or flowers of the field (Isa. 40:7–8; 1 Peter 1:24–25). "How frail is humanity! How short is life, and how full of trouble! Like a flower, we blossom for a moment and then wither. Like the shadow of a passing cloud, we quickly disappear" (Job 14:1–2). After we blossom, we wither, pass away, and are forgotten.

On the main corridor in my hospital is a bronze plaque from the year 1919, five feet wide and four feet tall, showing the picture of a doctor sitting in a chair smoking a cigar. Apparently he was once famous! But he has long since died. I have no idea who he was. I don't recognize his name. The plaque reminds me that nothing and no one lasts forever. If we get too attached to that which is passing away, it can be depressing. Human life is like that. Everywhere there are reminders of previous generations who have been forgotten, and reminders that you and I are next in line.

The basis for joy in the midst of all these wilting flowers and aging grasses is God, who is eternal. He is the foundation on which this book rests. God is the source of vitality and healing, the Author of life (Acts 3:15).

NOTES

Introduction

1. See Jeffrey H. Boyd, "A Biblical Theology of Chronic Illness," *Trinity Journal* 24 NS, no. 2 (Fall 2003): 189–206.

2. Catherine Hoffman, Dorothy Rice, and Hai-Yen Sung, "Persons with Chronic Conditions: Their Prevalence and Costs," *Journal of the American Medical Association* (*JAMA*) 276, no. 18 (Nov. 13, 1996): 1473–79. Their data came from the 1987 National Medical Expenditure Survey. This survey was later renamed the Medical Expenditure Panel Survey (MEPS), which is described at the website of the Agency for Healthcare Research and Quality: http://www.meps .ahrq.gov/WhatIsMEPS/Overview.HTM or www.ahrq.gov/data/mepsweb.htm.

3. Gerard F. Anderson and James R. Knickman, "Changing the Chronic Care System to Meet People's Needs," *Health Affairs* 20, no. 6 (Nov.–Dec. 2001): 146–60. Their data comes from the 1996 MEPS. The figure of 120 million comes from Exhibit 1 on p. 152 (see the large gray circle labeled "Any Chronic Condition"). It could be argued that this number (120 million) cannot be compared with the 90 million figure found by Hoffman, Rice, and Sung, because the studies used different diagnostic criteria. This issue is discussed in chapter 4. Partnership for Solutions was a research project funded by the Robert Wood Johnson Foundation and located at the Johns Hopkins University Bloomberg School of Public Health. Gerard Anderson was the principal investigator. Although their funding ended in September 2004, their website (www .PartnershipForSolutions.org) continues to be funded and should still exist.

4. Partnership for Solutions, *Chronic Conditions: Making the Case for Ongoing Care*, ed. Cynthia Anderson (Baltimore: Johns Hopkins University, 2002), 15. This book was downloaded from the website at www.partnershipforsolutions.org. This chartbook was updated in September 2004; however, the 2002 edition is used here.

5. Ibid., 8.

6. From the Centers for Disease Control, Chronic Disease Prevention and Health Promotion website at www.cdc.gov/wash ington/overview/chrondis.htm (Dec. 28, 2004).

7. C. S. Lewis, *Surprised by Joy* (New York: Harcourt Brace Jovanovich, 1984), 118.

8. Vicki A. Freedman and Linda G. Martin, "Contribution of Chronic Conditions to Aggregate Changes in Old-Age Functioning," *American Journal of Public Health* 90, no. 11 (Nov. 2000): 1755–60.

9. Vicki A. Freedman, Linda G. Martin, and Robert L. Schoeni, "Recent Trends in Disability and Functioning among Older

Adults in the United States: A Systematic Review," *JAMA* 288, no. 24 (Dec. 25, 2002): 3137–46.

10. H. Stephen Kaye, Mitchell P. LaPlante, Dawn Carlson, and Barbara L. Wenger, *Trends in Disability Rates in the United States, 1970–1994* (San Francisco: Disability Statistics Center, University of California San Francisco, 1996), abstract 17, figures 1 and 2 (available online at dsc.ucsf.edu/pub_listing.php?pub _type=abstract).

11. In the National Health Interview Surveys (NHIS) there is a decline only in IADLs (instrumental activities of daily living) but not for ADLs for the elderly. The National Long-Term Care Study (NLTCS) showed a decline in ADLs, IADLs, and other measures of disability among the elderly between 1982 and 1999.

12. Kenneth G. Manton, Larry Corder, and Eric Stallard, "Chronic Disability Trends in Elderly United States Populations: 1982–1994," *Proceedings of the National Academy of Sciences of the United States of America* 94, no. 6 (March 18, 1997), 2593–98; Burton H. Singer and Kenneth G. Manton, "The Effects of Health Changes on Projections of Health Service Needs for the Elderly Population of the United States," *Proceedings of the National Academy of Sciences of the United States of America* 95, no. 26 (Dec. 22, 1998): 15618–22; Kenneth G. Manton and XiLiang Gu, "Changes in the Prevalence of Chronic Disability in the United States Black and Nonblack Population above Age 65 from 1982 to 1999," *Proceedings of the National Academy of Sciences of the United States of America* 98, no. 11 (May 22, 2001): 6354–59; and Kenneth G. Manton, "Future Trends in Chronic Disability and Institutionalization: Implications for Long-Term Care Needs," *Health Care Manager* 3, no. 1 (June 1997): 177–91.

13. Partnership for Solutions, *Chronic Conditions*, 30.

14. Robert D. Abbott, Lon R. White, Webster Ross, Webster Ross, Kamal H. Masaki, J. David Curb, and Helen Petrovitch, "Walking and Dementia in Physically Capable Elderly Men," *JAMA* 292, no. 12 (Sept. 22/29, 2004): 1447–53; Jennifer Weuve, Jae Hee Kang, JoAnn E. Manson, Monique M. B. Breteler, James H. Ware, and Francine Grodstein, "Physical Activity, including Walking, and Cognitive Function in Older Women," *JAMA* 292, no. 12 (Sept. 22/29, 2004): 1454–61.

15. Michael E. McCullough, David B. Larson, W. T. Hoyt, et al., "Religious Involvement and Mortality: A Meta-Analytic Review," *Health Psychology* 19, no. 3 (May 2000): 211–22; Harold G. Koenig, J. C. Hays, David B. Larson, et al., "Does Religious Attendance Prolong Survival?: A Six-year Follow-Up of 3,968 Older Adults," *Journal of Gerontology, Series A—Biological Sciences and Medical Sciences* 54A, no. 7 (July 1999): M370–76; Robert A. Hummer, R. Rogers, C. Nam, and C. Ellison, "Religious Involvement and U.S. Adult Mortality," *Demography* 36, no. 2 (May 1999): 273–85; S. Bryant and W. Rakowski, "Predictors of Mortality among Elderly African Americans," *Research on Aging* 14, no. 1 (March 1992): 50–67; Norman Krause, "Stressors in Highly Valued Roles, Religious Coping, and Mortality," *Psychology and Aging* 13, no. 2 (June 1998): 242–55; M. Musick, J. House, and D. Williams, "Religion and Mortality in a National Sample" (paper presented at the annual meeting of the American Sociological Association, Chicago, 1999); William J. Strawbridge, Richard Cohen, Sarah Shema, and George A. Kaplan, "Frequent Attendance at Religious Services and Mortality over 28 Years," *American Journal of Public Health* 87, no. 6 (June 1997): 957–61; Douglas Oman and Dwayne Reed, "Religion and Mortality among the Community-Dwelling Elderly," *American Journal of Public Health* 88, no. 10 (Oct. 1998): 1469–75; T. E. Oxman, D. H. Freeman Jr., and E. D. Manheimer, "Lack of Social Participation or Religious Strength and Comfort as Risk Factors for Death after Cardiac Surgery in the Elderly,"

Psychosomatic Medicine 57, no. 1 (Jan.–Feb. 1995): 5–15; Christopher G. Ellison, Robert A. Hummer, Shannon Cormier, and Robert G. Rogers, "Religious Involvement and Mortality Risk among African American Adults," *Research on Aging* 22, no. 6 (Nov 2000): 630–67; Haltung King and Frances B. Locke, "American White Protestant Clergy as a Low-Risk Population for Mortality Research," *Journal of the National Cancer Institute* 65, no. 5 (Nov. 1980): 1115–24.

16. Walt Larimore, *Ten Essentials of Highly Healthy People* (Grand Rapids: Zondervan, 2003), 212.

17. Partnership for Solutions, *Chronic Conditions*, 30.

18. Gerard F. Anderson, "Physician, Public, and Policymaker Perspectives on Chronic Conditions," *Archives of Internal Medicine* 163, no. 4 (Feb. 24, 2003): 437–42.

19. Shin-Yi Wu and Anthony Green, *Projection of Chronic Illness Prevalence and Cost Inflation* (Santa Monica, CA: RAND Health Corporation, Oct. 2000, document # PM1144), 3–8, tables 1–10. The lower left corner of these tables gives the projected U.S. population and the number of people with no chronic illness, and those two numbers can be subtracted. The number of chronically ill used by Shin-Yi Wu and Anthony Green is from Partnership for Solutions, based on the 1996 MEPS. Population projections come from the Census Bureau.

20. Data from the National Health Interview Survey kindly provided by H. Stephen Kaye, director of research at the Disability Statistics Center at the University of California San Francisco in an email of January 8, 2004. These data are not age-corrected, because we are interested in the impact of the aging of the population, and age-correcting data hides from public view the impact of the aging of the population, an issue discussed at the end of chapter 4.

21. Kaye et al., *Trends in Disability Rates in the United States, 1970–1994*.

22. Edgar Sydenstricker, "The Vitality of the American People," in the *President's Research Committee on Social Trends: Recent Social Trends in the United States* (New York: McGraw Hill, 1933), figure 1 and table 1, 604–5; Marsha F. Goldsmith, "2020 Vision: NIH Heads Foresee the Future," *JAMA* 282, no. 24 (Dec. 22–29, 1999): 2287–90.

23. Hermann Brenner and Timo Hakulinen, "Are Patients Diagnosed with Breast Cancer before Age Fifty Years Ever Cured?" *Journal of Clinical Oncology* 22, no. 3 (Feb. 1, 2004): 432–38; Patricia A. Ganz, "Current Issues in Cancer Rehabilitation," *Cancer* 65, no. 3, suppl. (Feb. 1, 1990): 742–51.

24. "The prevalence of chronic illness or disability in adolescence has increased in recent years. In the past, children with certain chronic diseases did not reach adolescence, but over the last decade the survival rate has increased manyfold" (Mohammed Morad, Isack Kandel, Eytan Hyam, and Joav Merrick, "Adolescence, Chronic Illness and Disability," *International Journal of Adolescent Medicine and Health* 16, no. 1 (Jan.–Mar. 2004): 21–27.

25. "The Shape of Things to Come," *The Economist*, December 13, 2003: 11.

26. Scott M. Grundy, H. Bryan Brewer Jr., James I. Cleeman, Sidney C. Smith Jr., and Claude Lenfant, "Definition of Metabolic Syndrome: Report of the National Heart, Lung, and Blood Institute/ American Heart Association Conference on Scientific Issues Related to Definition," *Circulation* 109, no. 3 (Jan. 27, 2004): 433–38. The same article was also published in the journal *Arteriosclerosis, Thrombosis and Vascular Biology* 24, no. 2 (Feb. 2004): e13–e18.

Chapter 1 How to Survive

1. Augustine, *Confessions and the Enchiridion*, trans. Albert C. Outler (Philadelphia: Westminster, 1955), see *Enchiridion*, chap. 8, par. 27.

2. Dr. Russell Jaffe, Elisa/ACT Bio-technologies Labs, 14 Pidgeon Hill Drive, Suite 300, Sterling, VA 20165; 800-553-5472 (www.elisaact.com).

Chapter 2 A Survivor's Attitude

1. Information from the Quad Rugby website at www.quadrugby.com (Nov. 3, 2001).

2. Jacques Steinberg, "An Unrelenting Drive and a Harvard Degree," *New York Times*, May 17, 2000, A1.

3. Arthur Kleinman, *The Illness Narratives: Suffering, Healing, and the Human Condition* (New York: Basic Books, 1988), 137.

Chapter 3 Alternatives to Complaining

1. Norman Cousins, *Anatomy of an Illness as Perceived by the Patient* (New York: Bantam, 1991).

2. See Leland Ryken, James C. Wilhoit, and Tremper Longman III, eds., *Dictionary of Biblical Imagery* (Downers Grove, IL: InterVarsity, 1998), 409–10.

Chapter 4 Bad News and Good News about the Epidemic

1. Syden Stricker, "The Vitality of the American People."

2. Partnership for Solutions, *Chronic Conditions*, 11.

3. Gerard Anderson, "Testimony before the House Ways and Means Health Subcommittee, Hearing on Promoting Disease Management in Medicare" (April 16, 2002), downloaded from www.partnershipforsolutions.com/uploads/files/4_16_02_testimony.doc.

4. Wenke Hwang, Wendy Weller, Henry Ireys, and Gerard Anderson, "Out-of-Pocket Medical Spending for Care of Chronic Conditions," *Health Affairs* 20, no. 6 (Nov.–Dec. 2001): 267–78, data from p. 271, exhibit 1.

5. Ernest M. Gruenberg, "The Failures of Success," *Milbank Memorial Fund Quarterly— Health and Society* 55, no. 1 (Winter 1977): 3–24. Linda LeResche was a coauthor, but her name didn't get on the final paper because it started as a speech when Gruenberg won the Rema LaPouse award of the American Public Health Association.

6. Farley Mowat, *Never Cry Wolf* (Boston: Little, Brown, 1963), 124–25.

7. In December 2003, I downloaded the following PowerPoint slide from the Centers for Disease Control and Prevention website: www.cdc.gov/hiv/graphics/images/L207/L207-17.htm. I divided that graph into two charts (figures 3 and 4).

8. Andrew Coats, "Is Preventive Medicine Responsible for the Increasing Prevalence of Heart Failure?" *Lancet* 352, suppl. 1 (Aug. 1998): 39–41.

9. Vidya Bhushan, Nigel Paneth, and John L. Kiely, "Impact of Improved Survival of Very Low Birth Weight Infants on Recent Secular Trends in the Prevalence of Cerebral Palsy," *Pediatrics* 91, no. 6 (June 1993): 1094–1100.

10. As mentioned in note 2 of the Introduction, Catherine Hoffman used the National Medical Expenditure Survey. This survey was later renamed the Medical Expenditure Panel Survey (MEPS), which was and is conducted by those parts of the U.S. Government called the Agency for Healthcare Research and Quality and the National Center for Health Statistics. Its methodology is described at the website (www.ahrq.gov).

11. Hoffman, Rice, and Sung, "Persons with Chronic Conditions," 1473–79.

12. Anderson and Knickman, "Changing the Chronic Care System"; Hwang, Weller, Ireys, and Anderson, "Out-of-Pocket Medical Spending"; and Partnership for Solutions, *Chronic Conditions*.

13. Ihab Hajjar and Theodore A. Kotchen, "Trends in Prevalence, Awareness, Treatment, and Control of Hypertension in

the United States, 1988–2000," *JAMA*, 290, no. 2 (July 9, 2003): 199–206.

14. Anderson, "Physician, Public, and Policymaker Perspectives on Chronic Conditions," 437–42.

15. John K. Inglehart, "From the Editor: The Challenges of Chronic Disease," *Health Affairs* 20, no. 6 (Nov.–Dec. 2001): 7.

16. Institute of Medicine, *Crossing the Quality Chasm: A New Health System for the Twenty-First Century* (Washington, DC: National Academy Press, 2001).

17. Thomas Bodenheimer, Edward H. Wagner, and Kevin Grumbach, "Improving Primary Care for Patients with Chronic Illness," *JAMA* 288, no. 14 (Oct. 9, 2002): 1775–79; and Thomas Bodenheimer, Edward H. Wagner, and Kevin Grumbach, "Improving Primary Care for Patients with Chronic Illness: The Chronic Care Model," part 2, *JAMA* 288, no. 15 (Oct. 16, 2002): 1909–14.

18. Hoffman et al., "Persons with Chronic Conditions," 1473–79.

19. American Psychiatric Association, *Diagnostic and Statistical Manual*, 3d ed. (Washington, DC: American Psychiatric Press, 1987). Dr. Boyd's name appears in the Anxiety Disorders acknowledgments in the front. This book helped shape ICD-9.

20. A good example of the media message is the following article, which proposes that future breakthroughs in medicine will (paradoxically) decrease medical costs and benefit the American economy: Herbert Pardes, Kenneth G. Manton, Eric S. Lander, et al., "Effects of Medical Research on Health Care and Economy," *Science* 283, no. 5898 (1999): 36–37.

21. Jane Somerville, "Grown-Up Congenital Heart Disease: Medical Demands Look Back, Look Forward 2000," *Thoracic and Cardiovascular Surgeon* 49, no. 1 (Feb. 2001): 21–26; Bella Koifman, R. Egdell, and Jane Somerville, "Prevalence of Asymptomatic Coronary Arterial Abnormalities Detected by Angiography in Grown-Up Patients with Congenital Heart Disease," *Cardiology in the Young* 11, no. 6

(Nov. 2001): 614–18; Judith Therrien, Annie Dore, Welton Gersony, et al., "Canadian Cardiovascular Society Consensus Conference 2001 Update: Recommendations for the Management of Adults with Congenital Heart Disease, Part 1," *Canadian Journal of Cardiology* 17, no. 9 (Sept. 2001): 940–59; Judith Therrien, M. Gatzoulis, T. Graham, et al., "Canadian Cardiovascular Society Consensus Conference 2001 Update: Recommendations for the Management of Adults with Congenital Heart Disease, Part 2," *Canadian Journal of Cardiology* 17, no. 10 (Oct. 2001): 1029–50; Judith Therrien, C. Warnes, L. Daliento, et al., "Canadian Cardiovascular Society Consensus Conference 2001 Update: Recommendations for the Management of Adults with Congenital Heart Disease, Part 3," *Canadian Journal of Cardiology* 17, no. 11 (Nov. 2001): 1135–58.

22. Partnership for Solutions, *Chronic Conditions*, 15.

23. Wu and Green, *Projection of Chronic Illness Prevalence and Cost Inflation*, 17–23.

24. Partnership for Solutions, *Chronic Conditions*, 18.

25. Ibid., 30.

26. Wu and Green, *Projection of Chronic Illness Prevalence and Cost Inflation*, 17–23, tables 11–17.

27. Robert Pear, "Health Spending Rises to Record 15 Percent of Economy," *New York Times* 153 (Jan. 9, 2004): A1.

28. Karen Donelan, Robert J. Blendon, Craig A. Hill, et al., "Whatever Happened to the Health Insurance Crisis in the United States?: Voices from a National Survey," *JAMA* 276, no. 16 (Oct. 23–30, 1996): 1346–50.

29. Kenneth G. Manton and XiLiang Gu, "Changes in the Prevalence of Chronic Disability in the United States Black and Nonblack Population," data from table 2 on p. 6357.

30. Vicki A. Freedman and Linda G. Martin, "Understanding Trends in Functional Limitations among Older Ameri-

cans," *American Journal of Public Health* 88, no. 10 (Oct. 1998): 1457–62; Eileen Crimmins, Sandra Reynolds, and Yasuhiko Saito, "Trends in Health and Ability to Work among the Older Working-Age Population," *Journal of Gerontology, Series B—Psychological Sciences and Social Sciences* 54, no. 1 (Jan. 1999): S31–40; and Eileen M. Crimmins, Yasuhiko Saito, and Sandra L. Reynolds, "Further Evidence on Recent Trends in the Prevalence and Incidence of Disability among Older Americans from Two Sources: The LSOA and the NHIS," *Journal of Gerontology, Series B—Psychological Sciences and Social Sciences* 52, no. 2 (March 1997): S59–71.

31. John W. Rowe and Robert L. Kahn, *Successful Aging* (New York: Random House, 1998). The authors define the term *successful aging* on page 38. See also James F. Fries, "Successful Aging: An Emerging Paradigm of Gerontology," *Clinics in Geriatric Medicine* 18, no. 3 (Aug. 2002): 371–82.

32. James F. Fries, "Reducing Disability in Older Age: Editorial," *JAMA* 288, no. 24 (Dec. 25, 2002): 3164–66.

33. Freedman and Martin, "Understanding Trends in Functional Limitations among Older Americans," table 3, p. 1461; the data are age-adjusted.

34. Abbott et al., "Walking and Dementia in Physically Capable Elderly Men"; Jennifer Weuve et al., "Physical Activity, including Walking, and Cognitive Function in Older Women."

35. See the following studies: A. L. Dunn, M. H. Trivedi, J. B. Kampert, et al., "The DOSE Study: A Clinical Trial to Examine Efficacy and Dose Response of Exercise as Treatment for Depression," *Controlled Clinical Trials* 23, no. 5 (Oct. 2002): 584–603; J. W. Strawbridge, S. Deleger, R. E. Roberts, and G. A. Kaplan, "Physical Activity Reduces the Risk of Subsequent Depression for Older Adults," *American Journal of Epidemiology* 156, no. 4 (Aug. 15, 2002): 328–34; A. S. Mather, C. Rodriguez, M. F. Guthrie, et al., "Effects of Exercise on Depressive Symptoms in Older Adults with Poorly Responsive Depressive Disorder: Randomised Controlled Trial," *British Journal of Psychiatry* 180 (May 2002): 411–15; B. W. Penninx, W. J. Rejeski, J. Pandya, et al., "Exercise and Depressive Symptoms: A Comparison of Aerobic and Resistance Exercise Effects on Emotional and Physical Function in Older Persons with High and Low Depressive Symptomatology," *Journal of Gerontology, Series B—Psychological Sciences and Social Sciences* 57, no. 2 (March 2002): P124–32; A. M. Lane and D. J. Lovejoy, "The Effects of Exercise on Mood Changes: The Moderating Effect of Depressed Mood," *Journal of Sports Medicine and Physical Fitness* 41, no. 4 (Dec. 2001): 539–45; J. A. Blumenthal, M. A. Babyak, K. A. Moore, et al., "Effects of Exercise Training on Older Patients with Major Depression," *Archives of Internal Medicine* 159, no. 19 (Oct. 25, 1999): 2349–56; Andreas Broocks, B. Bandelow, G. Pekrun, et al., "Comparison of Aerobic Exercise, Clomipramine, and Placebo in the Treatment of Panic Disorder," *American Journal of Psychiatry* 155, no. 5 (May 1998): 603–9; G. A. Sachs, J. Rhymes, and C. K. Cassel, "Research Ethics: Depression and Mortality in Nursing Homes," *JAMA* 266, no. 2 (July 10, 1991): 215–16; E. W. Martinsen, A. Hoffart, and O. Solberg, "Comparing Aerobic with Nonaerobic Forms of Exercise in the Treatment of Clinical Depression: A Randomized Trial," *Comprehensive Psychiatry* 30, no. 4 (July–Aug. 1989): 324–31.

36. Richard G. Woodbury, "The Declining Disability of Older Americans," *Research Highlights in the Demography and Economics of Aging*, issue 5 (March 1999); downloaded (but no longer available) from the NIA Demography Centers website (http://agingmeta.psc.isr.umich .edu). See also "Disability Decline: What We Know and What We'd Like to Know," NIA-NBER Workshop Summary, Stone House, National Institutes of Health (Nov. 30, 2001),

downloaded December 28, 2004, from www.nia.nih.gov/NR/rdonlyres/AF0997F6 -0C16-4A76-96C0-D3780F00E6D4/3057/ disabilityworkshop1.pdf.

37. James F. Fries, "Measuring and Monitoring Success in Compressing Morbidity," *Annals of Internal Medicine* 139, no. 5, part 2, suppl. (Sept. 2, 2003): 455–59; James F. Fries, "Aging, Natural Death, and the Compression of Morbidity, 1980," *Bulletin of the World Health Organization* 80, no. 3 (2002): 245–50.

38. James Fries, email of February 23, 2004.

39. Fries, "Reducing Disability in Older Age: Editorial," 3164–66; and Vicki A. Freedman, Linda G. Martin, and Robert L. Schoeni, "Recent Trends in Disability and Functioning among Older Adults in the United States: A Systematic Review," 3137–46.

40. Fries, email of February 23, 2004.

41. Fries, "Reducing Disability in Older Age," 3164–66; and "Measuring and Monitoring Success in Compressing Morbidity," 455–59.

42. Stephen Kaye, email of March 2, 2004.

Chapter 5 The Value of Spiritual Resources

1. Ellen L. Idler, *Cohesiveness and Coherence: Religion and the Health of the Elderly* (New York: Garland, 1994).

2. Harold G. Koenig, *The Healing Power of Faith: How Belief and Prayer Can Help You Triumph over Disease* (New York: Simon and Schuster, 1999), 72–103, 262.

3. Stephen G. Post, Lynn G. Underwood, Jeffrey P. Schloss, and William B. Hurlbut, eds., *Altruism and Altruistic Love: Science, Philosophy, and Religion in Dialogue* (New York: Oxford University Press, 2002).

4. Peter H. VanNess, "Religious Rituals, Spiritually Disciplined Practices, and Health," in *Thinking Through Rituals: Philosophical Perspectives*, ed. Kevin Schilbrack (New York: Routledge, 2004), 251–72.

5. Kenneth I. Pargament, "Spiritual Coping with Chronic Illness," *Spirituality and Medicine Connection* 5 (Summer 2001): 1. This journal was published by David Larson's group, the International Center for the Integration of Health and Spirituality, but that group ceased to exist after Larson died, so the journal will probably be hard to obtain by interlibrary loan.

6. Kenneth I. Pargament, Harold G. Koenig, Nalini Tarakeshwar, and June Hahn, "Religious Struggle as a Predictor of Mortality among Medically Ill Elderly Patients: A Two-Year Longitudinal Study," *Archives of Internal Medicine* 161, no. 15 (Aug. 2001): 1881–85.

7. Harold G. Koenig, "An 83-Year-Old Woman with Chronic Illness and Strong Religious Beliefs," *JAMA* 288, no. 4 (July 24–31, 2002): 487–93.

8. Ellen L. Idler, Marc A. Musick, Christopher G. Ellison, et al., "Measuring Multiple Dimensions of Religion and Spirituality for Health Research: Conceptual Background and Findings from the 1998 General Social Survey," *Research on Aging* 25, no. 4 (July 2003): 327–65.

9. Data from the Center for Study of Global Christianity at the Gordon-Conwell Theological Seminary website (www .worldchristiandatabase.org), March 20, 2004, which presents the same statistics as David B. Barrett, George T. Kurian, and Todd M. Johnson, eds., *World Christian Encyclopedia: A Comparative Survey of Churches and Religions in the Modern World* (London: Oxford University Press, 2001).

10. Thich Nhat Hanh, *The Miracle of Mindfulness* (Boston: Beacon Press, 1999); and *Living Buddha, Living Christ* (New York: Riverhead Books, 1997).

11. From Reverend Koshu's home page (hometown.aol.com/reverendkoshu/index .htm) on March 15, 2004.

12. See Thich Nhat Hanh, *The Miracle of Mindfulness*.

13. Jon Kabat-Zinn, *Full Catastrophe Living: Using the Wisdom of Your Body and*

Mind to Face Stress, Pain, and Illness (New York: Bantam, 1990).

14. Somini Sengupta and Larry Rohter, "Where Faith Grows, Fired by Pentecostalism," *New York Times*, October 14, 2003, A1, A12. See tables at the end of the article on p. A12.

15. Jeffrey H. Boyd, "Theology of Chronic Illness" (paper presented at the 53d annual meeting of the Evangelical Theological Society, Colorado Springs, CO, Nov. 16, 2001). This manuscript is available by email at ETS@Zondervan.com, or online at www.tren.com. As Walter Unger says, there are many good ideas in that paper; however, be aware that I now see in retrospect that there are also two flaws in that paper. First, chronic illness should not be viewed as a curse from God. Second, my translation of the word *curse* in Revelation 22:3 is wrong. In Greek the sentence reads: "No longer will there be any cursed thing." A later revision of my thinking about the theology of chronic illness is published in *Trinity Journal* 24 NS, no. 2 (Fall 2003): 189–206, a paper that I still endorse.

16. Darrel W. Amundsen, "Medicine and Faith in Early Christianity," *Bulletin of the History of Medicine* 56, no. 3 (Fall 1982): 326–50, quote from p. 342.

17. Augustine, *On Patience*, section 11; John Chrysostom, *Homily 29 on Hebrews 12:4-6.*

18. Other writings of the Church Fathers on this subject can be found in the following: Augustine, *On Psalm 39*, verses 17–18; *On Psalm 77:2*, section 4; *Letter 38 to his brother Profuturus*, par. 1; John Chrysostom, *Homilies Concerning the Statues*, Homily 1, section 14; *Letters* 2 and 3 to Olympias; Jerome, *Epistle 38*, section 2.

19. Koenig, *Healing Power of Faith*, 255–75. Peter VanNess helped me develop the ideas in this chapter about the "unifying theory."

20. See Post, Underwood, Schloss, and Hurlbut, eds., *Altruism and Altruistic Love.*

21. Harold George Koenig, Michael E. McCullough, and David B. Larson, *Handbook of Religion and Health* (Oxford: Oxford University Press, 2001), 97–117; see chapter 6 on well-being.

22. Jeremy D. Kark, Galia Shemi, Yechiel Friedlander, et al., "Does Religious Observance Promote Health? Mortality in Secular versus Religious Kibbutzim in Israel," *American Journal of Public Health* 86, no. 3 (March 1996): 341–46.

23. Harold G. Koenig, L. K. George, H. J. Cohen, et al., "The Relationship between Religious Activities and Cigarette Smoking in Older Adults," *Journal of Gerontology, Series A—Biological Sciences and Medical Sciences* 53, no. 6 (Nov. 1998): M422–34; K. S. Kendler, C. O. Gardner, and C. A. Prescott, "Religion, Psychopathology, and Substance Use and Abuse: A Multimeasure, Genetic-Epidemiologic Study," *American Journal of Psychiatry* 154, no. 3 (March 1997): 322–29.

24. Koenig, *Healing Power of Faith*, 72–103, 262.

25. Although many people think the divorce rate among spiritual people is as high as that among the nonspiritual, a number of research studies indicate that spiritual people have stronger marriages and a lower divorce rate. See Koenig, McCullough, and Larson, *Handbook of Religion and Health*, 195–97; Koenig, *Healing Power of Faith*, 48–71; James McCarthy, "Religious Commitment, Affiliation, and Marriage Dissolution," in Robert Wuthnow, ed., *The Religious Dimension: New Directions in Quantitative Research* (New York: Academic Press, 1979), 179–97; Wesley Shrum, "Religion and Marital Stability: Change in the 1970s?" *Review of Religious Research* 21, no. 2 (Spring 1980): 135–47; Vaughn R. A. Call and Tim B. Heaton, "Religious Influence on Marital Stability," *Journal for the Scientific Study of Religion* 36, no. 3 (1997): 382–92.

Chapter 6 Christian Spiritual Resources

1. There are many translations of *The Way of a Pilgrim*. Here are a few: Helen Bacovcin, trans., *The Way of a Pilgrim* (San Antonio, TX: Image Press, 1985); Gleb Pokrovsky, trans., *The Way of a Pilgrim: Annotated and Explained* (Woodstock, VT: Skylight Paths, 2001); Dennis J. Billy, trans., *The Way of the Pilgrim: Complete Text and Reader's Guide* (Ligouri, MO: Ligouri Publications, 2000); R. M. French and Andrew Walker, trans., *The Way of a Pilgrim: A Classic of Orthodox Spirituality* (London: Society for Promoting Christian Knowledge, 1930); Gordon R. Dickson, trans., *The Way of the Pilgrim* (New York: Tor Books, 1999).

2. Albert S. Rossi, "Saying the Jesus Prayer," St. Vladimir's Orthodox Theological Seminary website, www.svots.edu/faculty (Oct. 19, 2003).

3. See also Igumen Chariton of Valamo, *The Art of Prayer*, trans. E. Kadloubovsky and E. M. Palmer (London: Faber and Faber, 1966).

4. Thomas E. Powers, *Invitation to a Great Experiment* (New York: Crossroad/Herder and Herder, 1990).

5. *Writings from the Philokalia on the Prayer of the Heart*, trans. E. Kadloubovsky and G. E. H. Palmer (London: Faber and Faber, 1967).

6. See note 15 of the introduction.

7. Koenig, Hays, Larson, et al., "Does Religious Attendance Prolong Survival?" Data come from figure 1, p. M373.

8. Ellen L. Idler and Stanislav V. Kasl, "Religion among Disabled and Nondisabled Persons II: Attendance at Religious Services as a Predictor of the Course of Disability," *Journal of Gerontology, Series B—Psychological Sciences and Social Sciences* 52B, no. 6 (Nov. 1997): S306–16.

9. For Arlene Pond's pamphlets or interviews with Ms. Pond, contact Maple Heights Baptist Church, 144 West Funderburg Road, Fairborn, OH 45324, 937-878-3333.

Chapter 7 Grab the Bull by the Horns

1. Larimore, *Ten Essentials of Highly Healthy People*, 212.

2. The unanimous U.S. Supreme Court decision in *Pegram vs. Herdrich* endorsed the idea that for twenty-seven years Congress promoted the formation of Health Maintenance Organizations and thereby endorsed "the profit incentive to ration care." See M. Gregg Bloche and Peter D. Jacobson, "The Supreme Court and Bedside Rationing," *JAMA* 284, no. 21 (Dec. 6, 2000): 2776–79. In June 2004 Justice Clarence Thomas, writing for the majority, reinforced that rationing by defending the Congressional legislation called *ERISA* in two Supreme Court cases, *Aetna Health Inc. vs. Davila*, no. 02-1845, and *Cigna HealthCare of Texas Inc. vs. Calad*, no. 03-83.

3. Inglehart, "From the Editor: The Challenges of Chronic Disease," 7.

4. David M. Eisenberg, Ronald C. Kessler, Cindy Foster, et al., "Unconventional Medicine in the United States: Prevalence, Costs, and Patterns of Use," *New England Journal of Medicine* 328, no. 4 (Jan. 28, 1993): 246–52. See also Ted J. Kaptchuk and David M. Eisenberg, "Varieties of Healing 1: Medical Pluralism in the United States," *Annals of Internal Medicine* 135, no. 3 (Aug. 7, 2001): 189–95; Ted J. Kaptchuk and David M. Eisenberg, "Varieties of Healing 2: A Taxonomy of Unconventional Healing Practices," *Annals of Internal Medicine* 135, no. 3 (Aug. 7, 2001): 196–204; David M. Eisenberg, Roger B. Davis, Susan L. Ettner, et al., "Trends in Alternative Medicine Use in the United States, 1990–1997: Results of a Follow-up National Survey," *JAMA* 280, no. 18 (Nov. 11, 1998): 1569–75.

5. See resources in the preceding note.

6. Richard Geiger, email of March 19, 2004.

7. Koenig, *Healing Power of Faith*, 119.

Chapter 8 The Wisdom of Caregivers

1. Partnership for Solutions, *Chronic Conditions*, 5, 30.

2. Institute for Health and Aging at the University of California San Francisco, *Chronic Care in America* (Princeton, NJ: Robert Wood Johnson Foundation, 1996), 62–63.

3. P. S. Arno, C. Levine, and M. M. Memmott, "The Economic Value of Informal Caregiving," *Health Affairs* 18, no. 2 (March–Apr. 1999): 182–88.

4. Carol Levine, "The Loneliness of the Long-Term Caregiver," *New England Journal of Medicine* 340, no. 20 (May 20, 1999): 1587–90.

5. University without Walls is sponsored by Dorot, a nonprofit organization affiliated with Caregivers' Connection in New York City. They can be contacted at www .dorotusa.org or by phone at 877-819-9147 or 212-769-2850.

Chapter 9 From Disabled to Is Able

1. The most popular secular books on this subject are Paul J. Donoghue and Mary Elizabeth Siegel, *Sick and Tired of Feeling Sick and Tired* (New York: W. W. Norton, 1994); and Stacy Taylor and Robert Epstein, *Living Well with a Hidden Disability* (Oakland, CA: New Harbinger, 1999).

2. Douglas Groothuis, "Seeing Invisible Disabilities," at www.gospelcom.net/ ivpress/groothuis/.

3. Patricia A. Fennell, *The Chronic Illness Workbook: Strategies and Solutions for Taking Back Your Life* (Oakland, CA: New Harbinger, 2001), 2.

4. Stephen Kaye, "Is the Status of People with Disabilities Improving?" (San Francisco: Disability Statistics Center, University of California San Francisco, 1998), abstract 17 (available online at dsc.ucsf .edu/pub_listing.php?pub_type=abstract).

5. Sherri and Wayne Connell's booklet, "Have a Little Faith!" is available through their website: The Invisible Disabilities Advocate at www.WhereIsGod.net.

6. Sherri L. Connell, "When Seeing Is *Not* Believing When Dealing with a Chronic Illness" at www.InvisibleDisabilities.com (Dec. 14, 2000).

7. Ibid.

8. Sherri L. Connell, "Where Is God?" at www.WhereIsGod.net (Dec. 2, 2003).

9. Ibid.

Chapter 10 Two Themes and Two Conclusions

1. From the Centers for Disease Control, Chronic Disease Prevention and Health Promotion website at www.cdc .gov/washington/overview/chrondis.htm (Dec. 28, 2004).

2. Jeffrey H. Boyd, "Tribute to an American Heroine" in Sherri Connell, *But You Look So Good*, reissued under the title, *Have a Little Faith*. This is available at the Connells' website "Where Is God?" at www .WhereIsGod.net/heroine.htm.

3. Koenig, *The Healing Power of Faith*, 29.

4. I used the following search request in the Logos Library System's computerized NIV Bible: "joy OR joyful OR joyous OR glad OR gladness OR happy OR happiness OR rejoice OR rejoices OR rejoiced OR rejoicing OR celebrate OR celebrated OR celebration OR celebrating OR delight OR delights OR delighted OR delightful" → 748 times in 596 Bible verses. When the words "praiseworthy OR praise OR praised OR praising" are added to the preceding request the computer finds these words used 1,151 times in 928 Bible verses.

5. Eleanor H. Porter, *Pollyanna* (London: Puffin Books, 1944), 193.

Jeffrey H. Boyd holds post-graduate degrees in theology, medicine, and chronic disease epidemiology. After receiving his M.Div. from Harvard University School of Divinity and serving briefly as an Episcopal priest, he went on to medical school and into the field of psychiatry. For the last twenty years he has served in a number of research and clinical positions and is currently chairman of behavioral health at the Waterbury Hospital Health Center, a Yale Medical School–affiliated teaching hospital.

Dr. Boyd has written dozens of both medical and theological journal articles and book chapters and is the author of *Reclaiming the Soul: The Search for Meaning in a Self-Centered Culture.* He is also active in the Evangelical Theological Society and Wheaton Theology Conference.

He and his wife, Maureen, live in Connecticut. For more information, visit his website at www.BeingSickWell.com.